EUROPE AGAINST CANCER

European Commission Series
for General Practitioners

Prepared for the Commission
of the European Communities
by the

European School of Oncology

Umberto Veronesi (Ed.)

Breast Cancer

Textbook for General Practitioners

With 10 Figures and 8 Tables

Springer-Verlag Berlin Heidelberg New York
London Paris Tokyo Hong Kong Barcelona

Professor Dr. Umberto Veronesi

Direttore Generale
Istituto Nazionale Tumori
Via Venezian 1, 20133 Milano, Italy

Warning: Neither the Commission of the European Communities nor any person acting on its behalf can accept responsibility for any use made of the information contained herein.

ISBN-13:978-3-540-53102-9 e-ISBN-13:978-3-642-76054-9
DOI: 10.1007/978-3-642-76054-9

2123/3145-543210 – Printed on acid-free paper

Foreword

The "Europe against Cancer" programme has, from its inception, emphasised the key role which general practitioners must play in the actions necessary to achieve its aim of reducing the incidence and the mortality from cancer in the European Community.
General practitioners, because of their day-to-day direct and continuing contact with patients, play a role not only in primary prevention and education of patients, but also in motivating their patients to accept secondary prevention and screening, some of it carried out by general practitioners themselves. These preventive activities are in addition to their traditional role in the care and management of patients with cancer at home, and increasingly, their role in active treatment.
In view of the importance of the general practitioner in the "Europe against Cancer" programme, the European Commission, with a view to providing general practitioners with up-to-date useful information, has sponsored the production of this series of publications on organbased cancers, especially written for general practitioners.

MICHEL RICHONNIER
Coordinator
of the "Europe against Cancer" programme,
Commission of the European Communities,
Brussels

Preface

The present textbook is the second in the series published by the Commission of the European Communities within the context of the "Europe Against Cancer" Programme. After lung cancer, it was felt that priority should be given to breast cancer, the most frequent neoplastic disease among European women.
The aim of these pages is to give a clear and at the same time complete and intensive information to the General Practitioner who has an important role, mainly in the early diagnosis of breast cancer, but also in other aspects of cancer care and treatment.
The textbook is composed of three sections: the first answering the key questions about the disease; the second dealing more in depth with the main aspects of diagnosis, treatment and rehabilitation; the third listing the main references on the subject.

UMBERTO VERONESI

Contents

First Part

Second Part

Editorial Board

HOW FREQUENT IS BREAST CANCER ?

Breast cancer is the commonest cancer among females in the countries of the European Community. The incidence of breast cancer within Europe varies from an annual, age-adjusted rate per 100,000 of 34.7 in Zaragoza (Spain) to the highest rate of 71.6 in Eindhoven in The Netherlands.

The highest rates are typically found in regions of Northern Europe - The Netherlands, Denmark, United Kingdom. Interestingly, the lowest breast cancer rates occur in the three cancer registration regions of Spain (Zaragoza, Navarra and Tarragona).

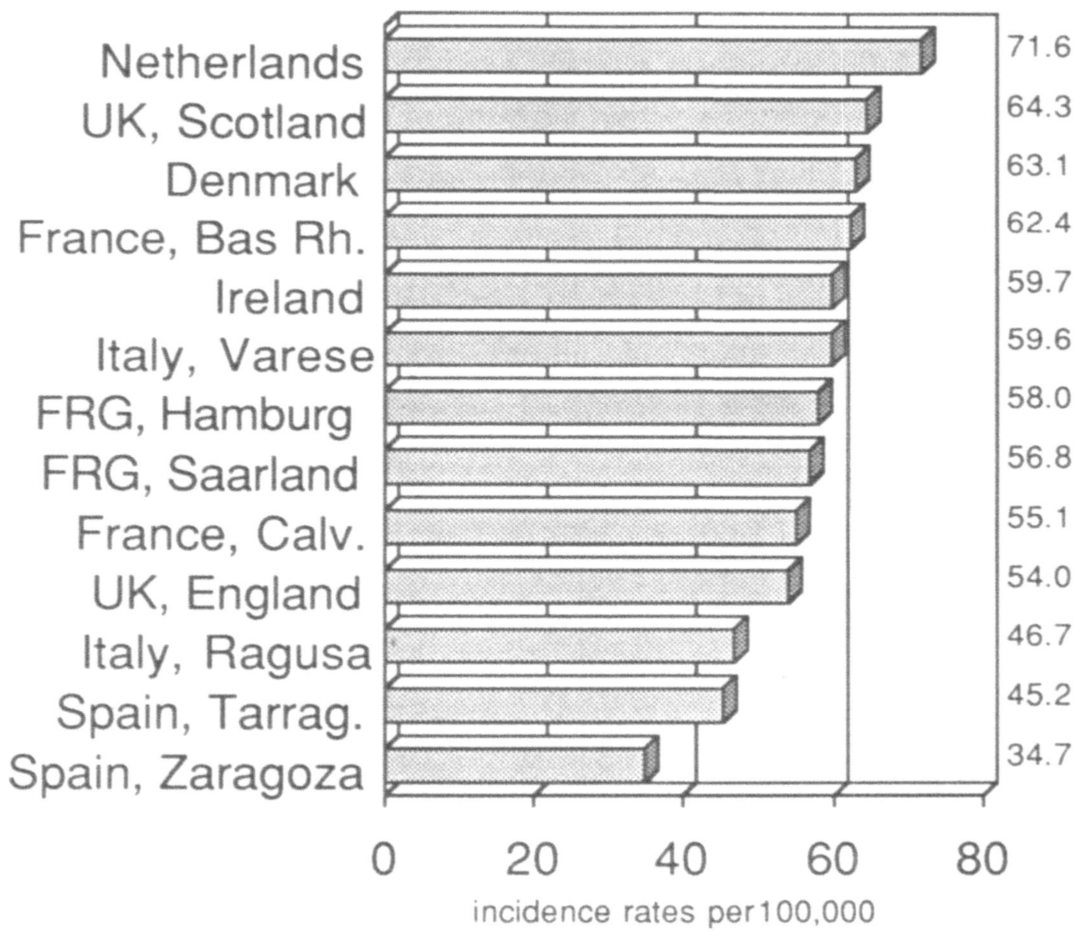

HOW MANY BREAST CANCER PATIENTS WILL DIE ?

The two-fold range of variation present in incidence rates within Europe is also found in national death rates. The highest age-adjusted death rate is found in the United Kingdom (28.5 per 100,000) and the lowest in Spain (13.7). Northern Europe (United Kingdom, Ireland, Belgium, The Netherlands, Denmark, Luxembourg and the Federal Republic of Germany) and Southern Europe (Italy, France, Portugal, Greece and Spain) are clearly demarcated as "high" and "low" breast cancer regions, respectively. Around the mid-1980s, over 60,000 women in the European Community died from breast cancer. Breast cancer deaths represented 15.0 per cent of all cancer deaths in women in Spain and 21.7 per cent of all cancer deaths in women in The Netherlands. Another way to express these data is that breast cancer represented the cause of 2.6 per cent of all deaths in women in Spain and 5.4 per cent of all deaths in The Netherlands. Other countries had intermediate levels.

Number of deaths for 100,000 women in EEC Countries.

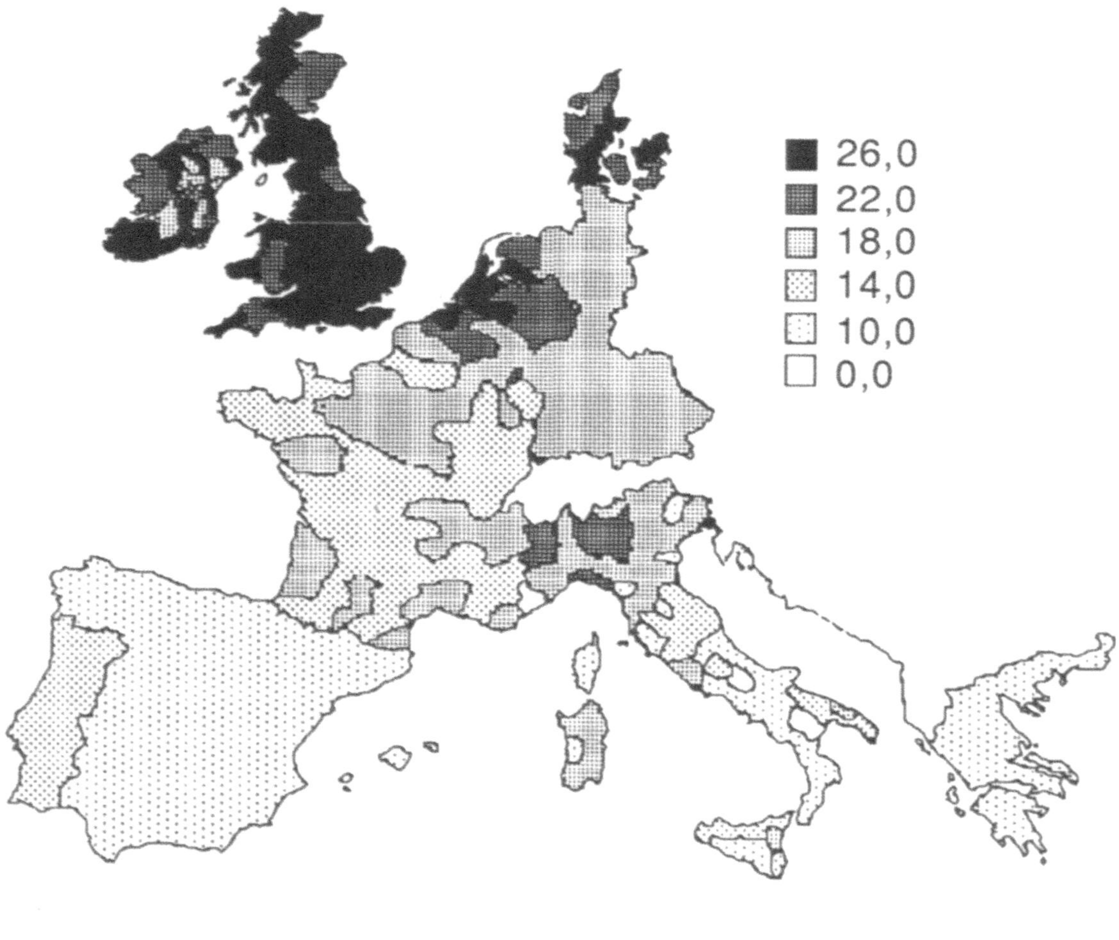

WHO IS AT RISK ?

There is a variety of breast cancer risk factors:

Age	100 times more common at age 70 than at age 30
Previous breast cancer	Confers an increased risk of a second primary cancer of the breast
Nulliparity	Nulliparous women have 50 per cent increased risk
Age at first birth	Women who have early age at first birth have a reduced risk of breast cancer
Parity	Increased parity decreases breast cancer risk
Artificial menopause	With bilateral oophorectomy, decreases risk
Breast feeding	May protect against premenopausal form of disease
Obesity	Increases risk at postmenopausal ages
Family history	If mother or sister has breast cancer, than risk increased mainly in premenopausal age groups
Radiation	Exposure to ionising radiation around menarche increases breast cancer risk
Benign breast disease	Increases the risk only if atypical dysplasia is present
Diet	Intake of saturated fat and / or total energy may increase the risk. Evidence that frequent vegetable consumption may decrease the risk

CAN THE RISK BE REDUCED ?

Primary Prevention

Avoidance of obesity may decrease risk of postmenopausal breast cancer, and switching from high-fat / low-vegetable diet to a lower-fat / higher vegetable diet may also contribute to a reduced risk.

Secondary Prevention

Screening by mammography may allow breast cancer to be diagnosed at an earlier stage than clinically possible and hence increase prospects for long-term survival.

Careful surveillance is required for some identifiable groups:

- Young women whose mother or sister has had breast cancer diagnosed before her menopause
- Women with benign breast disease recorded as atypical dysplasia
- Women who survive previous breast cancer or ovarian cancer

WHAT ARE THE MEANS OF DETECTION ?

The vast majority of breast cancers are detected casually by the patient herself. This does not constitute early detection as over two thirds of cases are already more than 2 cm. in diameter and more than half show histologically involved axillary nodes. Physical examination (breast self examination) and mammography are the tests presently available for breast cancer detection.

Breast Self Examination (BSE)

When regularly and properly performed, may identify breast cancer at an early stage, that is when both cure and conservative surgery are possible. Women should be encouraged to perform regular BSE but they should also be correctly informed about the limits of this procedure. BSE is poorly specific and most of the abnormalities reported by the woman actually will turn out to be benign. BSE may miss breast cancer, especially small lesions, and the negative outcome of this procedure should not be completely reassuring. BSE should not be an alternative to screening. If the latter is possible BSE should be performed in the interval between two consecutive screening controls.

Physical Examination (PE)

Is currently performed with the aim of breast cancer detection. Nevertheless PE is not very accurate in the detection of early breast cancer. PE will miss most cancers less than 1 cm in diameter (or even larger especially when deeply located in large breasts). Since accurate predictive signs of cancer are lacking in most cases the criteria adopted for clinical suspicion are relatively non specific. Many suspicious lesions on PE will turn out to be benign. Thus any abnormality on PE should undergo further diagnostic work up.

Mammography (M)

Is the most accurate test presently available for breast cancer detection. Tumour size affects the sensitivity of M less than it does for PE, and preclinical detection of minimal cancers is possible. Indeed the sensitivity of M to detect cancer lesions is often strongly reduced by the radiological density of the juvenile breast. The usefulness of M as a detection tool for breast cancer in healthy women depends mainly on age. The cutoff age most commonly advised for its use in screening is 50 years.

HOW USEFUL IS SCREENING ?

Breast cancer may be detected in its more favourable asymptomatic resectable stages both by physical examination (PE) and mammography (M). Mammography is by far more sensitive, especially in older women, allowing the detection of subclinical cancer. Several studies have been conducted to assess the value of systematic population screening, age being the only risk indicator employed. Mammography has been always employed whereas physical examination has been employed only in a few studies. All studies reporting long term mortality data showed a reduction in breast cancer mortality in the screening group with respect to non screened controls. This reduction was statistically significant over the age 49 whereas no convincing reduction has been observed thus far in women age 40-49. Presently available data do not allow the assessment of the role of physical examination in addition to mammography and the optimal rescreening interval (1, 2 or 3 years). Large-scale mammographic screening for early breast cancer in asymptomatic women can be advocated as a public health policy in women over the age 49. Further investigation is needed to define the optimal screening protocol although biennial mammography seems to be the most reasonable option at this time.

Reduction of mortality by screening (randomized trials only, age > 49):

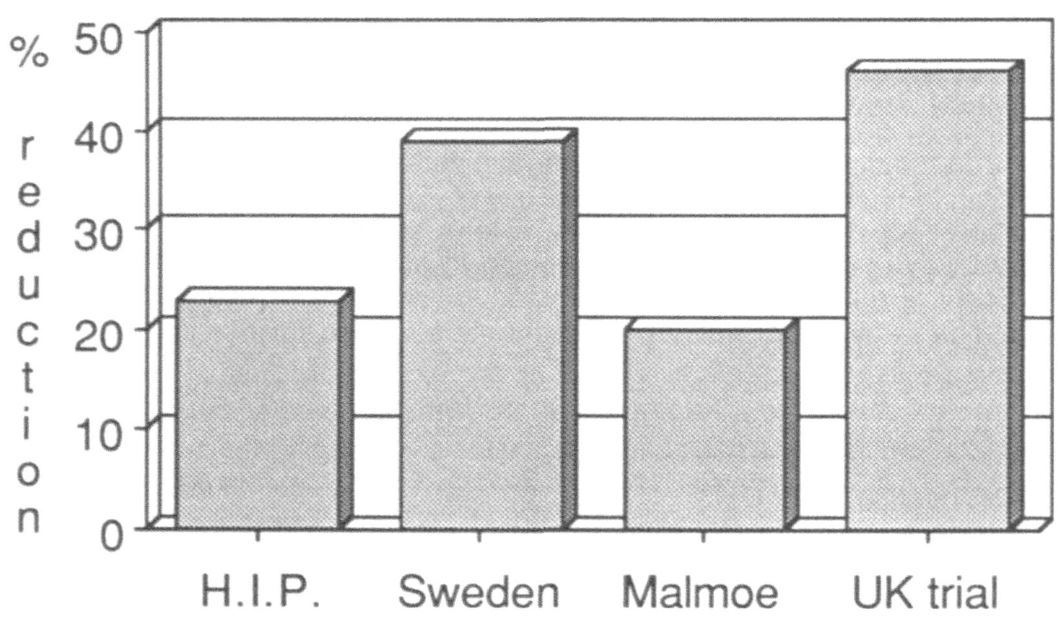

ARE BENIGN NODULES PREMALIGNANT ?

- An increased risk of developing breast cancer with respect to the normal population has been claimed for several benign conditions, but most of these statements are not supported or are refuted by convincing scientific evidence.

- As a matter of fact the majority of cancers occur in women with no other benign lesion and the majority of women presenting with a benign lesion of the breast will never develop breast cancer.

- No prediction of increased risk of developing breast cancer should be made on the basis of solely clinical evidence, as is often suggested in the presence of a clinical diagnosis of fibrocystic disease.

- The relative risk of subsequent breast cancer is substantially that of the normal population for almost all histologically assessed benign lesions (lipoma, fibroadenoma, cyst, different types of dysplasia, intraductal papilloma) with the sole exception of atypical ductal or lobular hyperplasia (relative risk = 5:1). Atypical hyperplasia is a rare condition accounting for about 1% of all benign biopsies. Even in these cases the adopted measures for breast cancer prevention should not exceed periodic screening recommendations.

- As a general rule surgical biopsy of breast abnormalities should be aimed only at cancer diagnosis, not at identifying high risk benign lesions. Benign biopsies should never be regarded as a benefit. Women with benign lesions should be firmly reassured and should not be advised any selective follow up.

WHAT ARE THE SYMPTOMS ?

The greater majority (over 95%) of patients with breast cancer are subjectively symptomatic at the time of detection. Symptoms of breast cancer can be caused by local, metastatic or remote effects of the disease, although symptoms at detection are due to local growth in all but very few cases. A breast lump is by far the most common and the only symptom. Other less frequently encountered symptoms include bloody discharge from the nipple, nipple retraction or deviation, dimpling, infiltration or ulceration of the skin overlying the tumour and enlarged ipsilateral axillary nodes. Unfortunately the most common symptoms (lump, dimpling of the skin, bloody discharge) are not specific for cancer. For example, the majority of breast lumps are due to benign lesions. Any woman presenting with these symptoms should be suspected of having breast cancer and should undergo further diagnostic work up. Non bloody nipple discharge or breast pain, which are frequent symptoms in self referring women, are quite aspecific and not significantly associated with cancer. Metastatic or remote effects are usually absent at the time of first diagnosis.

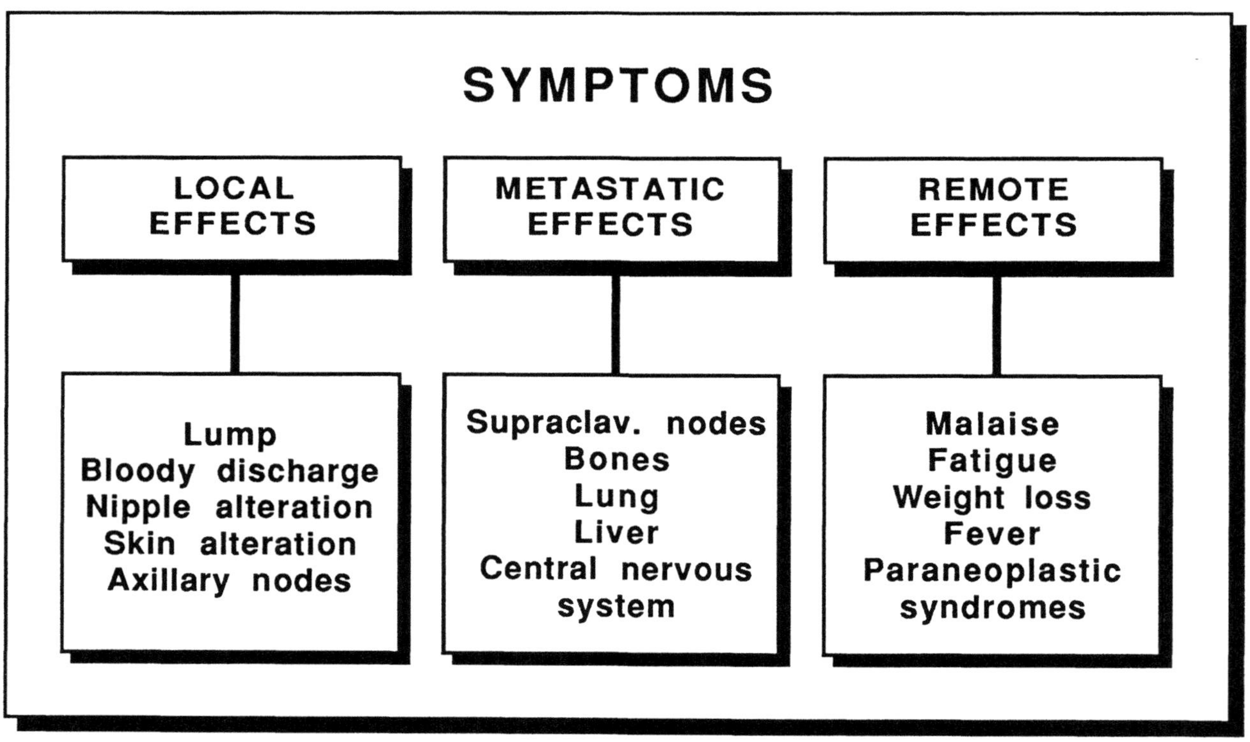

WHAT ARE THE INITIAL STEPS IN DIAGNOSIS ?

The procedures applied to establish the diagnosis of breast cancer obviously vary according to the clinical presentation. The initial examination in patients suspected of having breast cancer should always include physical examination and mammography followed by fine needle aspiration, or nipple discharge cytology in selected cases. Additional diagnostic procedures, such as sonography, galactography or pneumocystography, may be optionally performed in dubious cases, although there is no convincing evidence that they actually improve the cumulative accuracy of physical examination, mammography and cytology. A combined diagnostic approach is illustrated in the following chart.

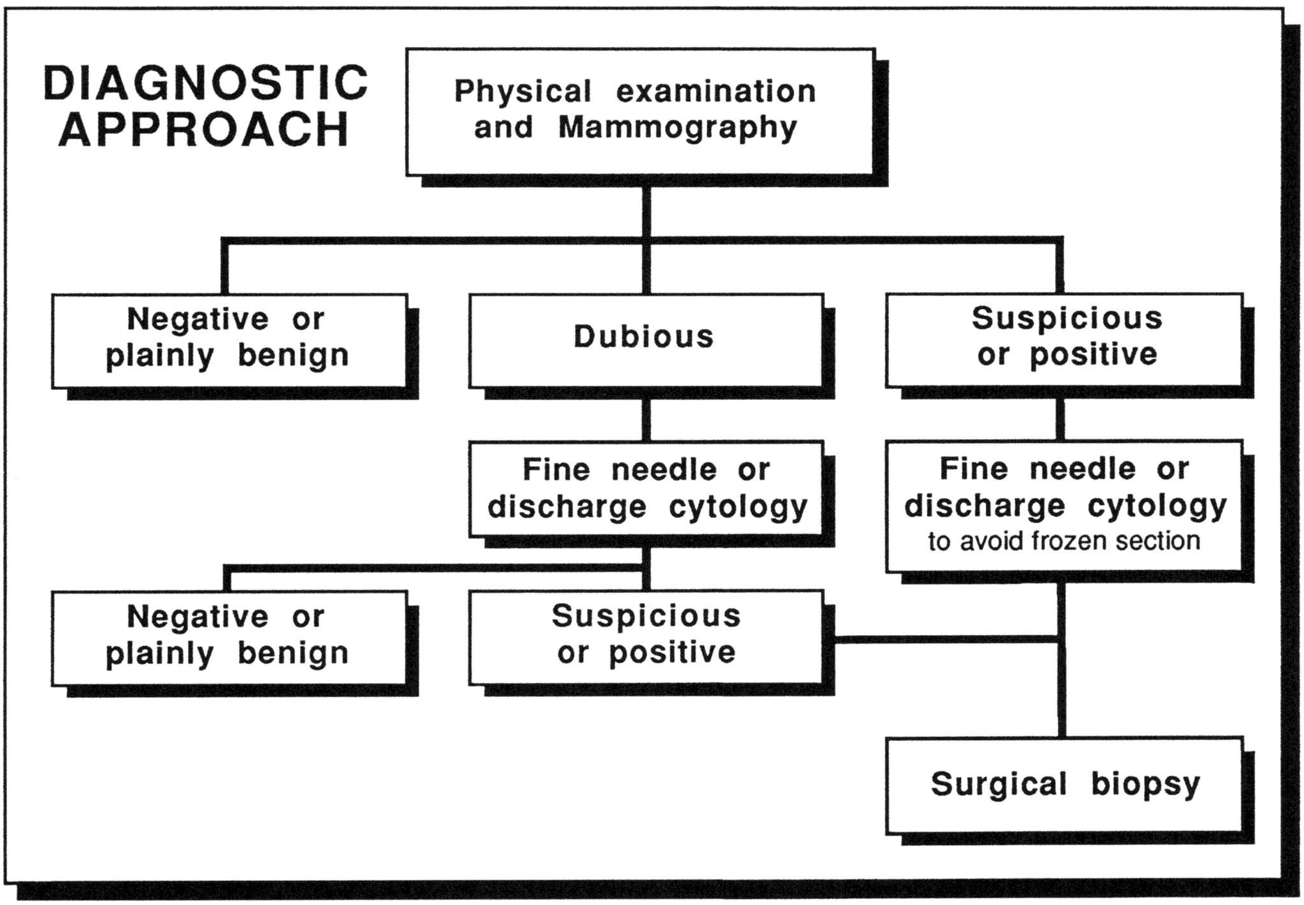

WHAT IS THE RELEVANCE OF NON-INVASIVE CARCINOMAS ?

- ❑ In spite of their name ductal carcinoma in situ (DCIS, intraductal carcinoma) and lobular carcinoma in situ (LCIS, lobular neoplasia) must be regarded as benign conditions.

- ❑ Their non-infiltrating condition excludes locoregional or distant spread and cure is achieved in 100% of cases by local control.

- ❑ Progression to infiltrating carcinoma after biopsy alone is far from being systematic (20%) in LCIS, which is often multicentric and even bilateral. Simple follow up after surgical excision is most commonly recommended.

- ❑ Total mastectomy is most commonly recommended for DCIS because of the risk of multicentricity or of progression to infiltrating cancer. Conservative surgical options are increasingly advocated for lesions of limited size.

- ❑ Detection of DCIS or LCIS should not necessarily be regarded as of benefit. Although infiltrating cancer may be prevented in some cases, overdiagnosis of non-progressing, non-life-threatening cases cannot be excluded, especially in screening programmes which increase the detection rate of these lesions.

WHAT ARE THE MOST IMPORTANT PROGNOSTIC FACTORS ?

Tumour size and histologically assessed nodal involvement are commonly considered the fundamental prognostic indicators in breast cancer. Attribution to Stages I-III (UICC-TNM System) is based only on these two variables.

Although tumour size and nodal status are strictly correlated, an independent prognostic significance of each factor is evident. The classic distinction between involved (N+) and non involved (N-) nodes provides only a rough estimate of the expected prognosis. In fact, the number of involved nodes seems a much more reliable prognostic index. An independent prognostic significance has been denied for many other factors, such as sex, age, race, tumour site, menstrual status. A significant prognostic correlation has been reported for other factors, such as histological grading, hormonal receptor content and, more recently, mitotic activity (labelling index), the latter being presently the more promising. Nevertheless literature evidence on these factors is either controversial or too limited and further research is needed.

At the present time and in current clinical practice, none of the proposed indicators seems to predict prognosis better than the combination of nodal involvement and tumour size.

10 year survival according to T and N categories:

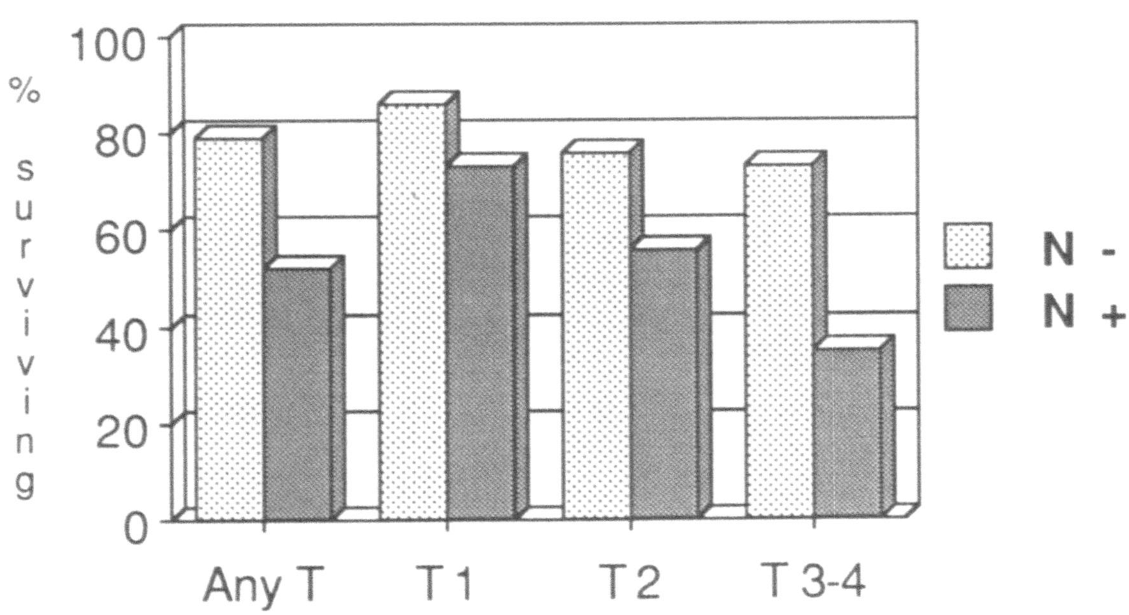

WHAT TYPE OF SURGERY?

- During the last few decades surgical treatment of breast cancer has undergone considerable modification due largely to changes in concepts concerning the natural history of breast cancer, to a progressive reduction in the size of the cancer detected today in comparison with the past and to improved surgical (ablative and reconstructive) and radiotherapeutic techniques.

- Small carcinomas: (less than 2-3 cm in diameter) the procedure followed is generally that of breast-preserving techniques. Lumpectomy: removal of the primary carcinoma together with a limited margin of normal tissue (1 cm), without removing any of the overlying skin. Quadrantectomy: removal of an entire quadrant of the breast with excision of the corresponding cutaneous area. The latter provides a better local control than the simple lumpectomy. With both techniques, postoperative radiotherapy should be applied. Axillary dissection is performed simultaneously.

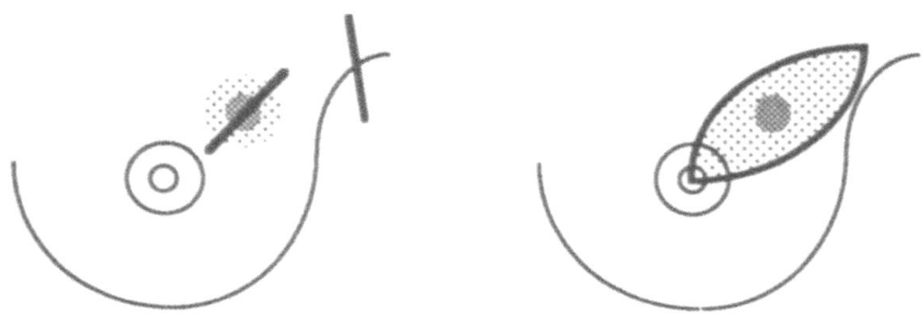

lumpectomy quadrantectomy

- Larger carcinomas: (more than 2-3 cm in diameter) the procedure of choice is generally mastectomy and total axillary dissection. Present techniques spare the major pectoralis muscle and often the minor pectoralis muscle as well.

- The traditional Halsted mastectomy, in which both pectoralis muscles are removed "en bloc" with the axillary nodes, is performed today only in exceptional cases of extensive tumours invading the muscular structures with massive invasion of the axillary nodes and in cases of locally advanced tumours after chemotherapy and/or radiotherapy, as a salvage mastectomy.

- Other types of more extensive operations, such as mastectomy with removal of the internal mammary nodes and superradical mastectomy, are performed even more rarely.

WHAT ARE THE RESULTS OF SURGERY ?

The overall results of breast cancer treatment can, today, be considered as satisfactory. Considering the total number of cases seen in a Western European Hospital, we can observe a ten-year survival of between 50% and 60% of all cases. But if we consider only the cases with small carcinomas of the breast (less than 2 cm in diameter), which represent roughly 40% of all diagnosed cases, the ten-year survival comes close to 80%. This finding underlines the importance of the early detection of breast cancer in achieving high levels of curability. Apart from the size of the primary tumour, there are other factors which influence survival. The most important factors are axillary metastases, the growth rate and the hormonal receptor status. As regards axillary invasion, survival is inversely proportional to the number of involved nodes with a very poor prognosis when more than 10 lymph nodes are metastatic. The rate of oestrogen and progesterone receptors in the cancer cells is important for prognosis. When both oestrogen (ER) and progesterone (PR) receptors are present the prognosis is good, whilst their absence is an unfavourable sign. Other prognostic factors are the pathological grade, thymidine labelling index, the ploidy and the oncogene amplification which, however, are infrequently used as routine values. From the pathological point of view, apart from infrequent, well-differentiated tumour types (papillary, medullary, colloid, tubular) with a good prognosis, it is important to mention that ductal and lobular in situ carcinomas have 100% cure rates.

Survival by number of positive axillary nodes:

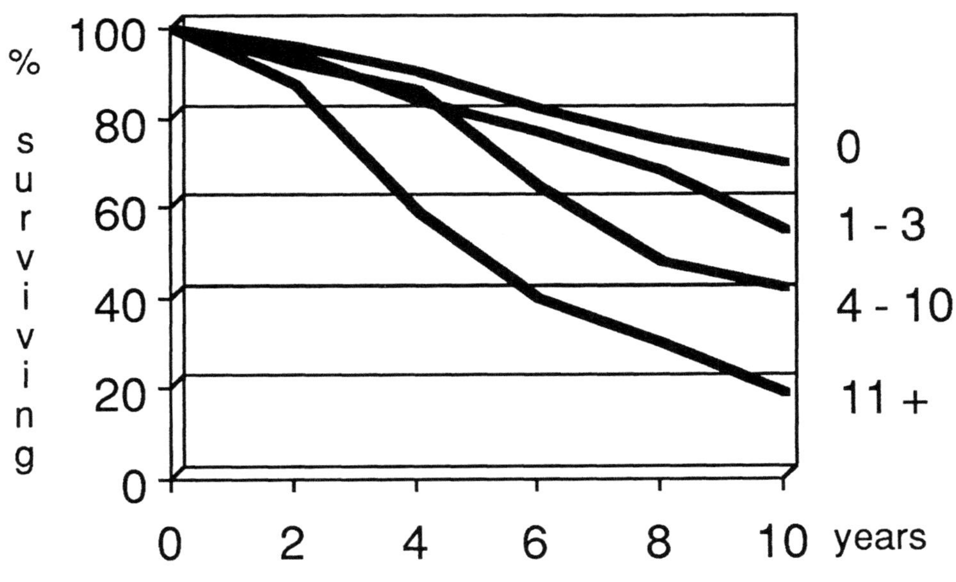

WHICH PATIENTS SHOULD RECEIVE RADIOTHERAPY FOR BREAST CANCER ?

Localised, "Operable" disease

- ❑ **Irradiation of the breast:**
  For small lesions, in breast conserving treatment : after quadrantectomy or lumpectomy, the breast is irradiated to sterilize residual microscopic disease, limiting the incidence of local recurrences.

- ❑ **Irradiation of the thoracic wall:**
  For large lesions after mastectomy : in **some** patients with a high risk of local recurrence (large tumours, multiple positive nodes, non radical resection) an irradiation of the thoracic wall is carried out.

- ❑ **Irradiation of regional lymph nodes:**
  In the treatment of regional lymph nodes radiotherapy is seldom indicated. It can be used for treatment of the axilla, although usually surgical axillary clearance is carried out. The treatment of the parasternal nodes, if deemed necessary, is nowadays always done with radiotherapy. Radiotherapy of the lymph nodes contributes to locoregional control. It has little or no effect on survival as the patient group with positive nodes is also prone to distant metastases.

Inoperable disease

- ❑ Radiotherapy to the breast and the regional lymph nodes, high doses are necessary for locoregional control.

Metastatic disease

- ❑ Important palliative role of irradiation for some metastatic locations such as bone, skin, lymph node or brain metastases.

- ❑ Radiotherapy on the primary tumour and nodal localisations only for palliative indications. Low doses can often be used when the course of the disease can be expected to be relatively short.

WHAT IS THE BENEFIT OF RADIOTHERAPY ?

- Radiotherapy is a local treatment agent. This means it will only kill tumour cells within the volume encompassed in the radiation beams. The radiation doses which are required to exterminate clinical tumour masses can only be given over limited parts of the body. Radiotherapy can thus only be expected to be effective as a curative agent in situations where the tumour is potentially still in a localised stage. In all other cases, where distant localisations are known to exist, the use of radiotherapy has to be assessed on its impact on the course of the disease by partial tumour eradication. This is a palliative effect: for instance, locoregional control in an otherwise metastasised patient.

- It has to be understood that a number of factors predict for high incidences of local recurrences in the breast or the thoracic wall and the regional lymph nodes. The most important ones are the size of the tumour and the invasion of axillary nodes. However, the same factors do also affect the chance of distant metastases.

- Selecting patients with a high risk of local recurrence, one always ends up with groups having high frequencies of distant metastases. Effect on survival can only be expected in the small group of patients where local tumour was left after surgery, but where still no distant (micro)metastases existed.

- Prevention of local relapses has been proven to be much more effective than treatment as only about half of the clinically apparent masses can be controlled. A relapse after insufficient therapy may be the cause of unnecessary prolongation and possible dissemination of tumour activity.

WHO IS A CANDIDATE FOR SYSTEMIC THERAPY ?

- Systemic therapy is a treatment given to a patient on the assumption that it will have a generalized effect upon occult metastatic disease.
- Results from randomized trials conducted during the past 2 decades show that some form of systemic adjuvant therapy reduced both relapse and mortality of breast cancer. These reductions were significant but of modest magnitude. Their extrapolation for patient-care purposes are relevant only for patients with an increased risk of relapse (those with involved axillary nodes; some with node-negative disease).
- Patients should be treated within the framework of clinical trials aimed at improving the results of therapy.

Systemic treatments shown to be effective are:

Premenopausal	Combination chemotherapy for 6 courses e.g., cyclophosphamide, methotrexate and 5-fluorouracil (CMF)
Postmenopausal	Endocrine treatment with tamoxifen for a duration of two or more years (or until relapse).

WHAT ARE THE SIDE EFFECTS OF SYSTEMIC THERAPY ?

Endocrine therapy (tamoxifen)

Generally very well tolerated. Hot flushes and gastric discomfort are the most frequent side effects. Nausea and vomiting might occur after beginning treatment, but usually regress spontaneously without discontinuation of therapy. Other rare side effects include: vaginal bleeding, lassitude, headache, leg cramps, dizziness, water retention with peripheral oedema, and diarrhoea. If used in premenopausal women: might induce ovulation (patient should be informed).

Chemotherapy (CMF)

Cyclophosphamide can be given orally on days 1-14 of a 28-day course, with methotrexate and 5-fluorouracil given intravenously on days 1 and 8 of the same course. The CMF combination can also be given entirely i.v. once every 3 weeks. Side effects are common and in most cases can also be treated to improve tolerance. These include nausea, vomiting (in the majority of the patients from mild to moderate; severe only in very few patients), epigastric pain, alopecia, stomatitis, and diarrhoea. Antiemetic therapy must be administered in a regular fashion from start of therapy to minimize anticipatory nausea and vomiting. Stomatitis and diarrhoea should be carefully monitored because they represent a contra-indication for the administration of methotrexate and 5-fluorouracil. Bone marrow suppression and its consequences are predictable and the nadir for white cell count in peripheral blood is usually between the 9th and the 28th day, with full recovery at the beginning of the fifth week, when the subsequent course starts. It is essential that counts and history of side effects be done on the day of a scheduled i.v. drug administration, to avoid unpredicted risk of severe toxicity. Conjunctivitis requiring medication is occasionally observed. Tiredness during therapy weeks is common. Amenorrhoea is seen in about 70% of the patients receiving a CMF combination chemotherapy. Responsible for this is an ovarian insufficiency due to the drugs (cyclophosphamide). Amenorrhoea-related symptoms are difficult to treat because of the contraindication for the use of steroid hormone replacement therapy in these patients.

HOW TO TREAT OVERT METASTATIC DISEASE ?

With few exceptions, the patient with overt metastases will die of, or with, the disease. Help her learn how to live with the disease. Aim to obtain maximal palliation with minimal side effects. Knowledge of the course of the disease is essential for treatment choice and for guidance of the patient. Use clinical (disease-free interval - DFI), extent of metastases) and biochemical (steroid hormone receptors in the tumour) parameters to choose therapeutic approach:

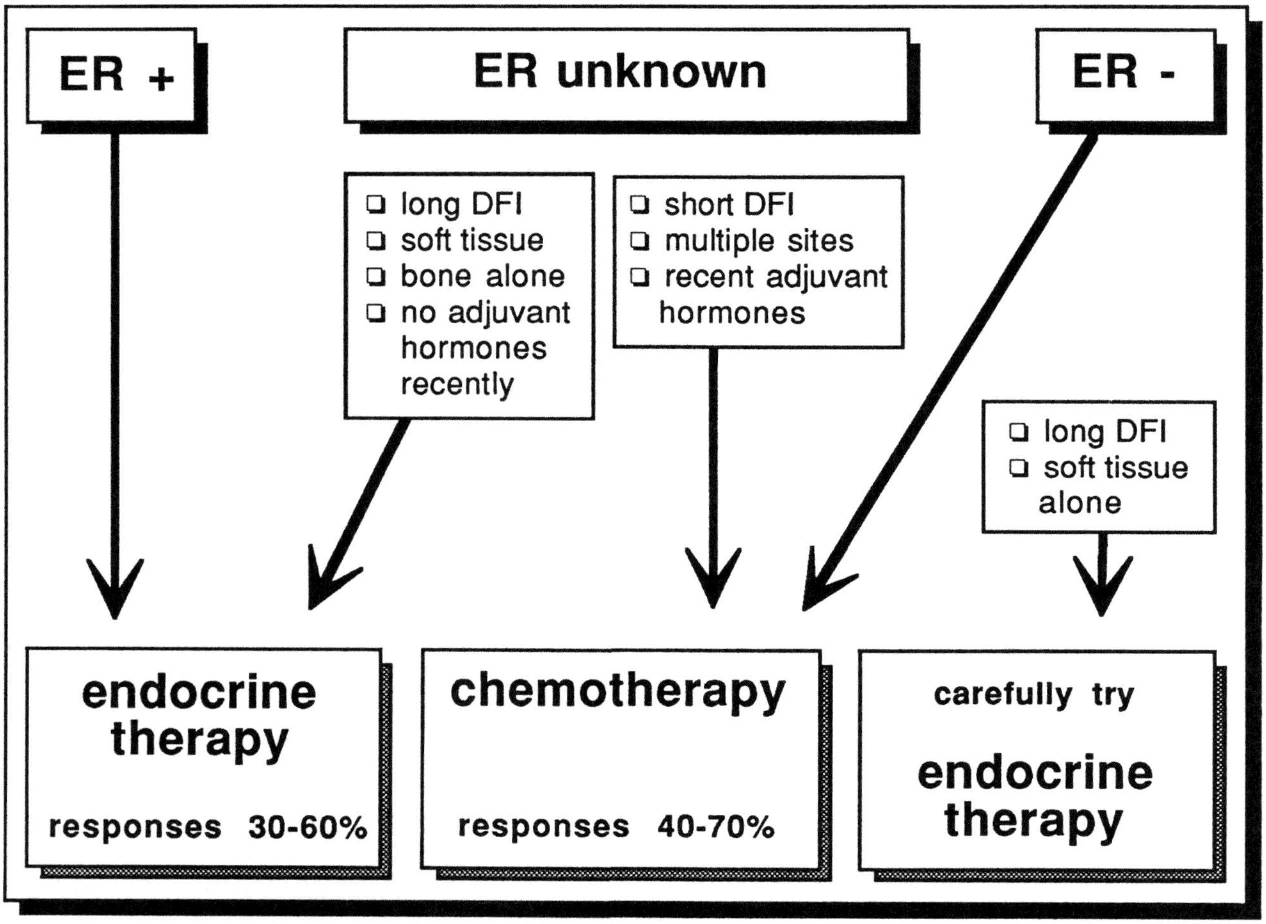

Secondary treatment choice is based upon previous response. Many special situations require specific interventions: local recurrence, ipsilateral and contralateral breast, bone alone, CNS involvement, spinal cord compression, malignant effusions.

HOW TO SUPPORT THE TERMINAL PATIENT ?

The co-existence of many factors which interact require a simultaneous therapeutic intervention to achieve:

- ❑ Control of specific symptoms (e.g., nausea, vomiting, epilepsy)
- ❑ Control of pain
- ❑ Relief of anxiety
- ❑ Reduction of the impact of general symptoms (e.g., tiredness, depression)

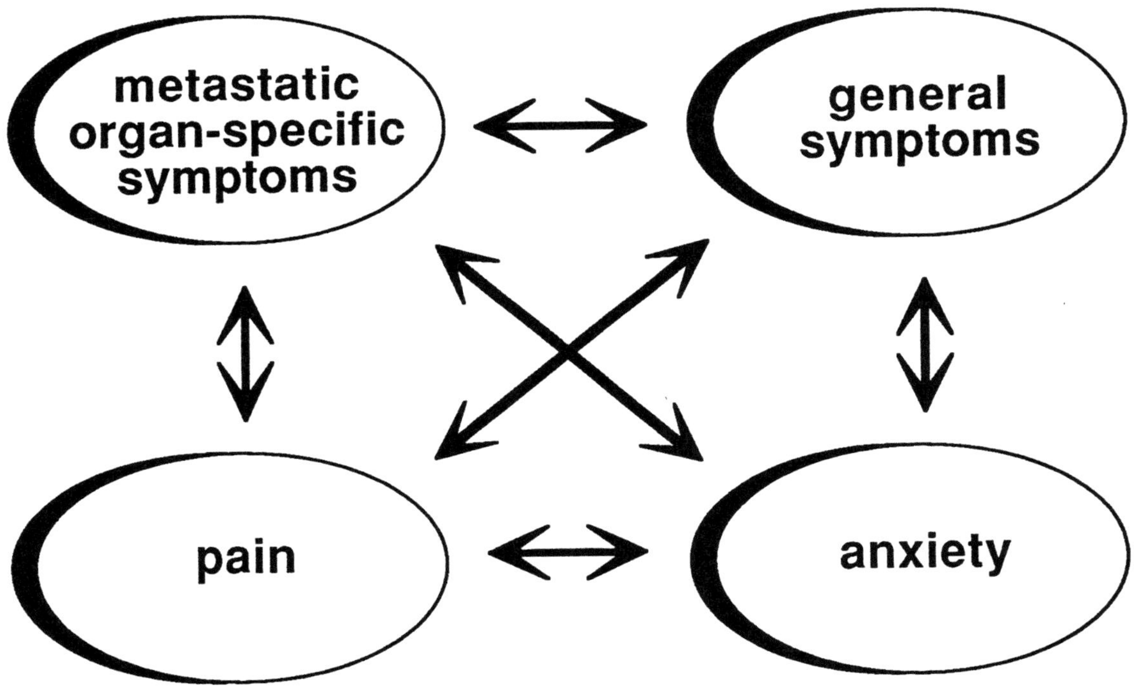

Keep in mind:

- ❑ Supportive care requires constant feedback
  This is essential for any of the steps, especially pain control
- ❑ Pain control might require systemic treatment (do not forget constipation) as well as regional approaches or surgical intervention
- ❑ Encourage social / family support

Epidemiology of Breast Cancer

It was estimated that in 1980 there were over 500,000 new cases of breast cancer first diagnosed in women throughout the world, and that in the three decades subsequent to 1950, breast cancer caused the deaths of nearly one million women in the United States alone. Within the 12 Member States of the European Economic Community (EEC), the number of deaths attributed to breast cancer rose from 30,695 in the mid-1950s to 60,965 per annum in the mid-1980s: almost a doubling of the cases.

There were also substantial rises in each one of the Member States in the age-adjusted rate per 100,000, the percentage of all cancer deaths in women attributed to breast cancer and the percentage of all deaths attributable (Table 1).

Table 1. Breast cancer mortality in EEC Countries: comparison 1955 and 1985

	1955			1985		
	Number	SRW (1)	% Cancer (2)	Number	SRW (1)	% Cancer (2)
UK Scotland	838	22.0	16.4	1,253	27.4	17.8
N. Ireland	177	19.6	15.4	308	27.6	20.0
England	8,495	23.7	19.7	13,513	29.3	20.4
Ireland (3)	313	17.5	15.0	554	25.7	18.0
Belgium (3)	1,304	18.8	14.4	2,269	25.9	19.9
Netherlands	1,426	23.8	18.1	3,052	26.5	21.7
Denmark	729	24.2	17.1	1,263	27.6	18.2
Luxembourg (4)	67	22.0	16.2	95	30.0	21.4
Germany	5,827	15.4	12.0	13,701	22.4	16.8
Italy (5)	4,115	13.6	13.8	9,570	20.3	17.9
France	5,091	14.4	12.8	9,313	19.0	18.0
Portugal	523	10.4	13.3	1,236	16.6	17.5
Greece (6)	241	4.8	6.3	1,195	15.1	16.8
Spain (7)	1,549	8.2	9.1	3,644	13.7	15.0

(1) Standardised mortality rates on the world population; (2) % of all cancer deaths; (3) data for 1984 used; (4) 1967 earliest year available; (5) data for 1983 used; (6) 1961 earliest year available; (7) data for 1960 and 1981 used

Descriptive Epidemiology

The highest mortality rates for breast cancer in the EEC are found in the United Kingdom (28.5 per 100,000 per annum), Ireland (26.5), Belgium (26.2), The Netherlands (26.1), Denmark (26.0) and Luxembourg (25.1). Rates are slightly lower in the Federal Republic of Germany (21.5), Italy (19.7) and France (19.1). The lowest mortality rates are recorded in Portugal (15.6), Greece (15.1) and Spain (13.7). Thus, there is an approximate two-fold variation in breast cancer mortality among Member States of the EEC (Fig. 1).

This same two-fold range in the variation is seen in incidence rates of breast cancer recorded among those areas in the European Economic Community covered by cancer registration schemes and whose data were published in the most recent volume of "Cancer Incidence in Five Continents".

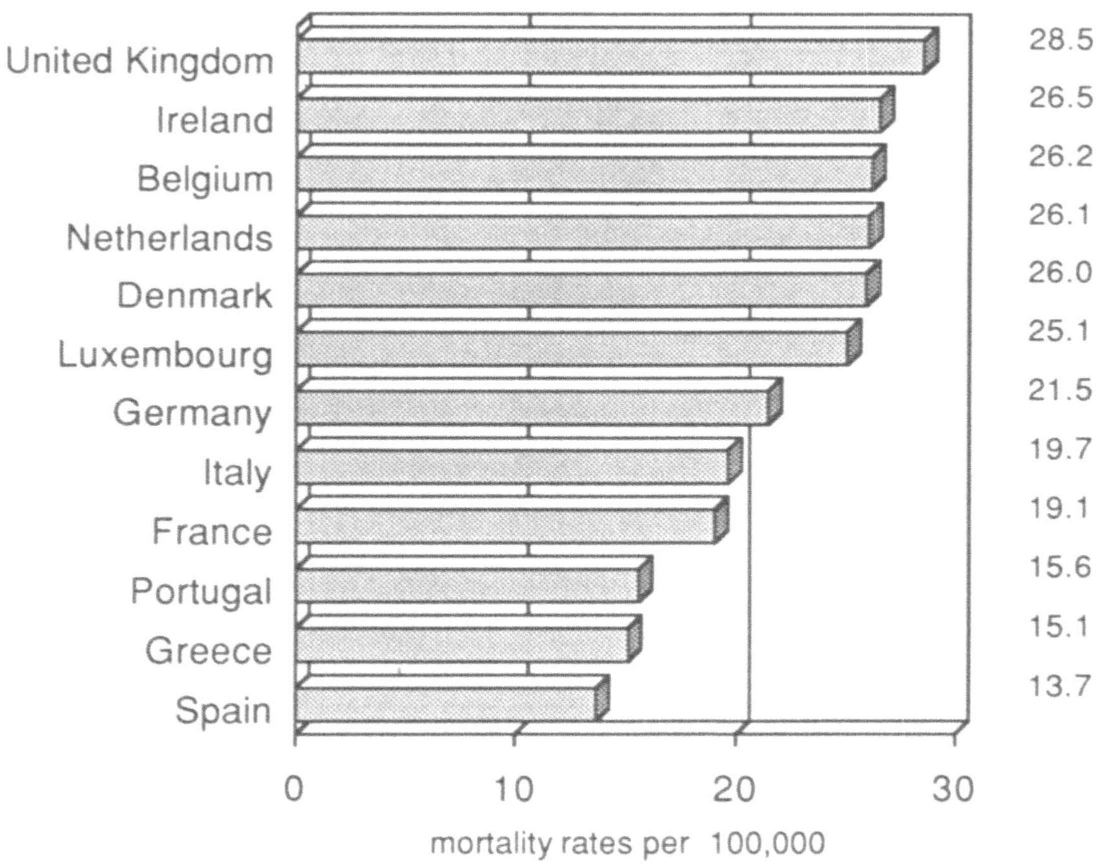

Fig. 1. Average annual age-standardised mortality rates per 100,000 for breast cancer among females in cancer registry regions of the European Economic Community (1980-1984)

The highest incidence rates were recorded in Eindhoven in The Netherlands (71.6), South East Scotland (64.3) and Denmark (63.1). Interestingly, the lowest rates recorded were found in the three cancer registration regions of Spain; Tarragona (45.2), Navarra (38.7) and Zaragoza (34.7) (Fig. 2).
In international terms, breast cancer rates in the EEC are amongst the highest recorded. Breast cancer represents over one-quarter of all incident cases of cancer in women (excluding non-melanoma skin cancer) not only in Northern EEC countries (United Kingdom, The Netherlands, Federal Republic of Germany) but also in Latin countries (Italy, France, Spain). These figures are similar, perhaps very slightly lower, than those found in Canada (29.1%) and among Whites in the United States (27.9), but are slightly higher than corresponding figures in Nordic countries (Sweden, Norway, Finland, Denmark) (23.5%).

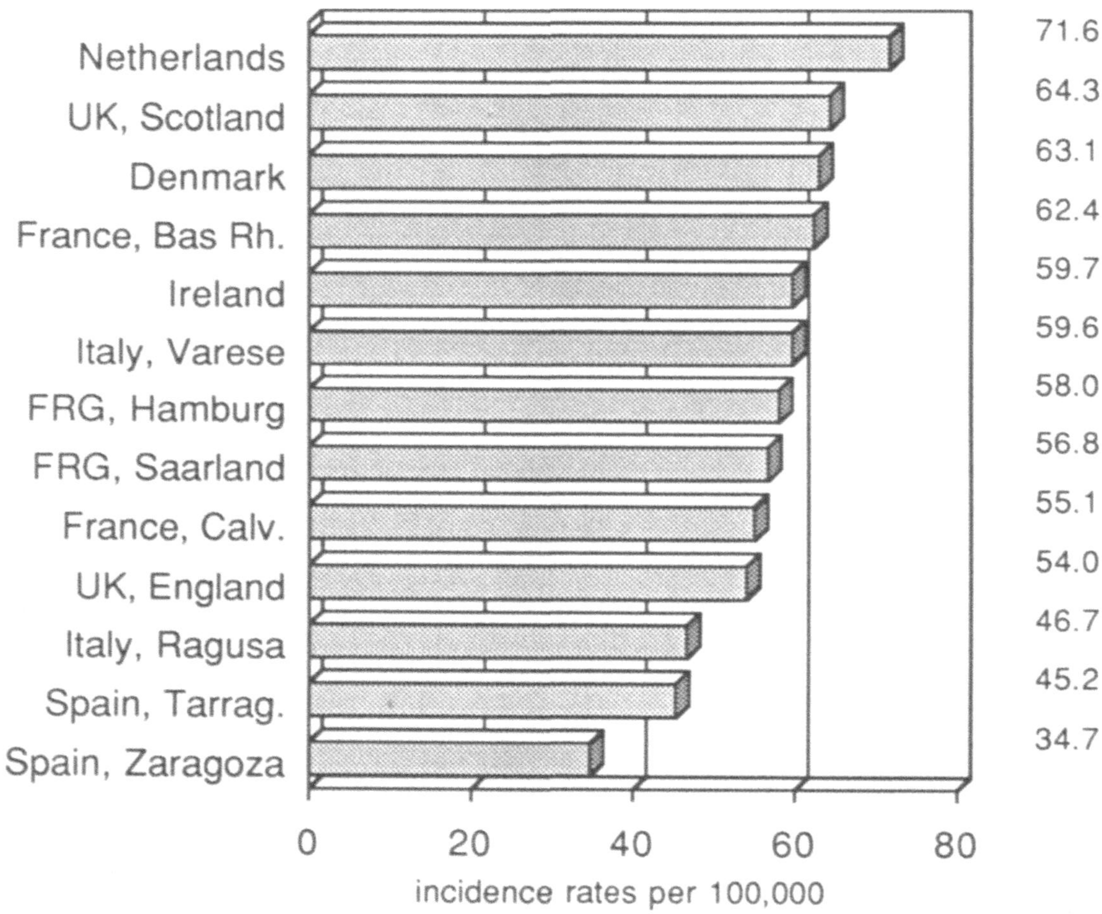

Fig. 2. Average annual age-standardised incidence rates per 100,000 for breast cancer among females in cancer registry regions of the European Economic Community (1978-1982)

Time trends

Table 1 clearly shows the overall increase which has taken place in breast cancer mortality in EEC countries. However, such cross-sectional data can easily mask important changes taking place among birth cohorts. This is certainly the case for breast cancer in Europe. In France (Fig. 3), it is clear that there is no interruption in the continuing pattern of increase taking place among successive birth cohorts. Similar patterns are to be found in the data from Italy, the Federal Republic of Germany, Portugal and Greece.

On the other hand, there appears to be stabilisation or indeed some evidence of downward trends among younger birth cohorts (those born since the 1930s and 1940s) in The Netherlands (Fig. 4). Similar patterns to this are to be found from the data from the United Kingdom, Ireland, Belgium and Denmark. Thus, it is clear from this disparity that rates of breast cancer in Europe will continue to come together over future decades.

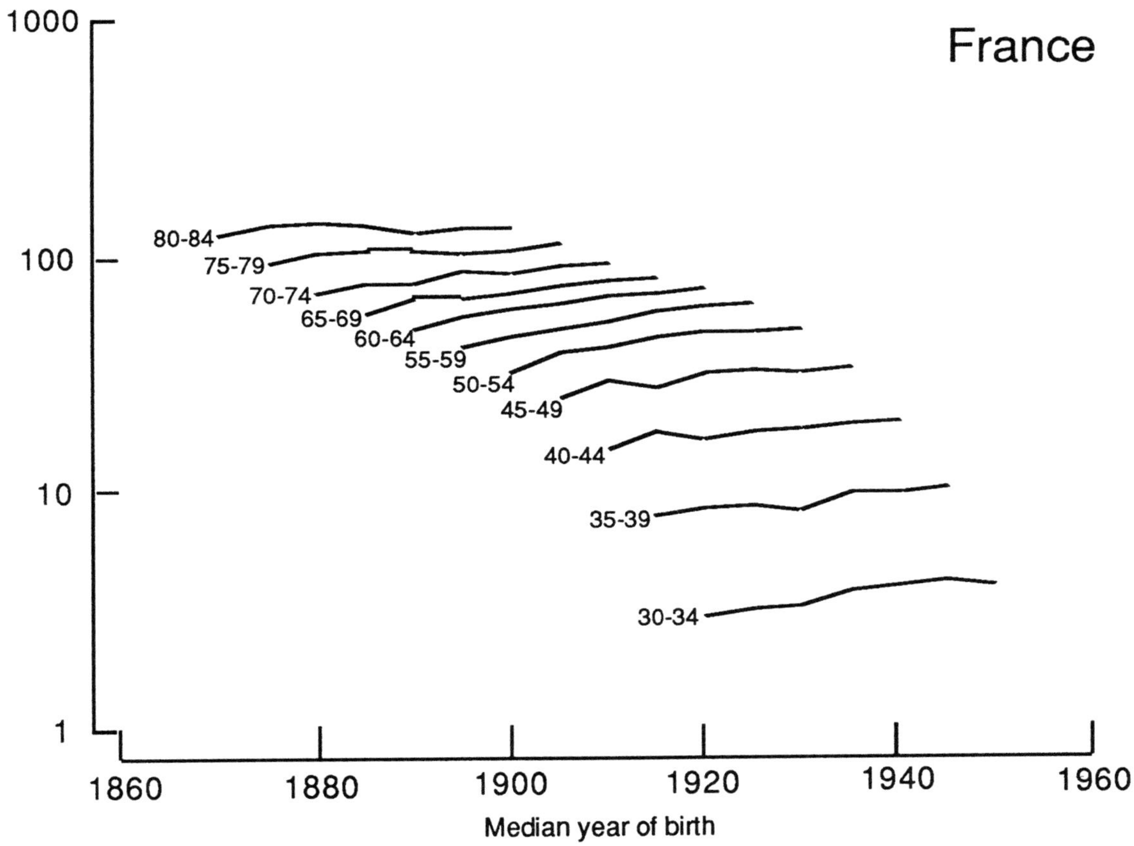

Fig. 3. Age-specific mortality rates from breast cancer in France (1955-1984), presented by age and median year of birth

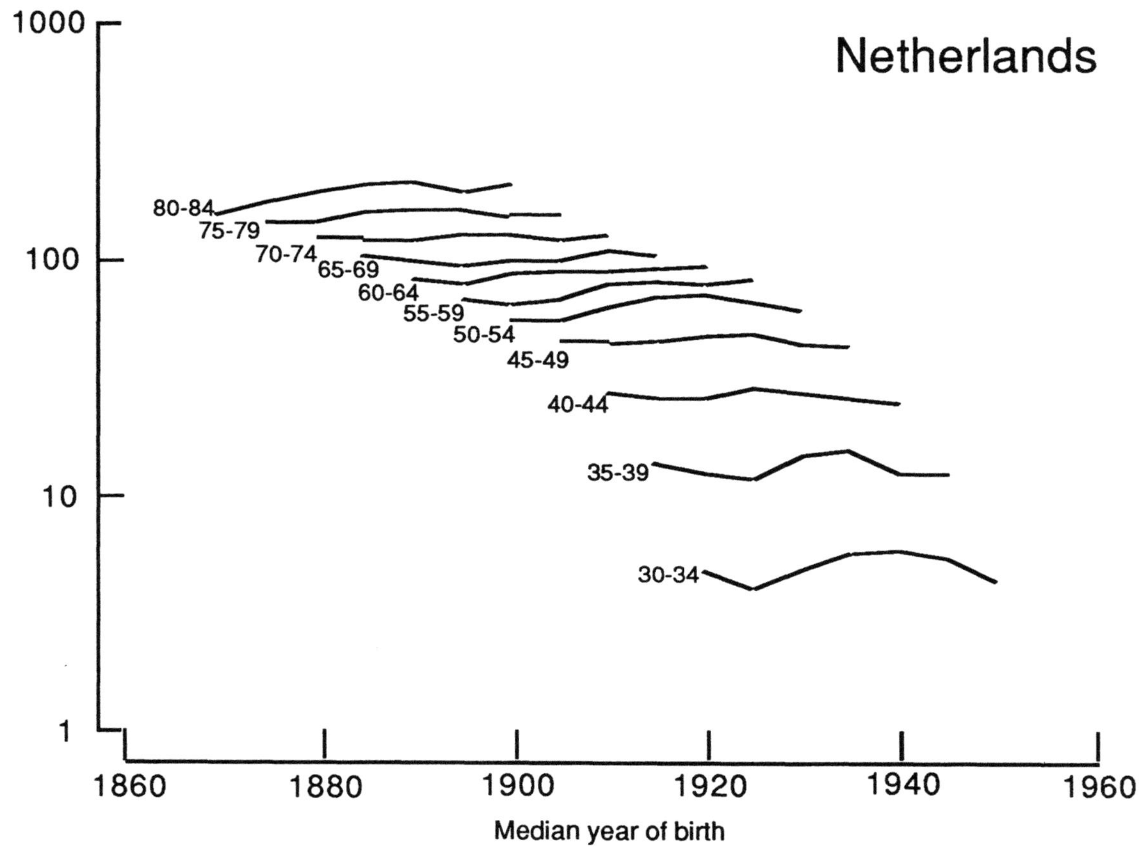

Figure 4. Age-specific mortality rates from breast cancer in The Netherlands (1955-1984), presented by age and median year of birth

An interesting trend in incidence is apparent in Nordic countries. Hakulinen investigated the Nordic data in depth and found that risk among birth cohorts has been increasing in all Nordic countries at postmenopausal ages. However, the authors noted that the risk for those born in the 1920s and the 1930s was the same although these groups had only been observed at pre-menopausal ages at the time of the study. MacMahon reported a levelling off in risk among cohorts of women in Connecticut born since 1925 and suggested that the future trend was worth watching in view of the possibility that the overall breast cancer rates could level off or decline. Similarly, using data up until 1984, it has been shown that the risk of breast cancer among younger cohorts of women in Scotland has been declining. A declining mortality rate from breast cancer in young women in the United States has also been reported; this was contrary to the pattern expected following delays in childbearing which started in the 1960s. In contrast, however, White reported a 22% increase in breast cancer incidence in women aged 25-44, resident in Washington State between 1974-1977 and 1982-1984. These findings are similar to the increase of 27% observed in breast cancer incidence between 1972 and 1981 among women aged 30-39 in Sweden. A report of incidence data in England and Wales demonstrated increases for all ages but smaller rises among young women than among old women. The situation regarding trends in breast cancer among younger women is obviously not consistent throughout the world and the data from all SEER registry areas (Cancer Registration regions of the United States) do not show any increase in breast cancer incidence in women under the age of 45.

In summary, there are many hints emerging from several populations that the rate of increase in breast cancer risk in younger cohorts of women is slowing down, or even falling. It is a situation which requires verification in other population groups not yet investigated and one which merits continual surveillance.

Variation in Breast Cancer Incidence by Personal Characteristics

The large international variation in the incidence and mortality from breast cancer demonstrated above could reflect variation in genetic predisposition to breast cancer, or it could support hypotheses of environmental causation. Data exist to compare breast cancer occurrence among members of the same community according to characteristics such as socioeconomical status, residence, race and religion. Boyle demonstrated the consistently higher levels of breast cancer in whites than in blacks in five cancer registry regions of the United States based on data covering 1973-1977 (Table 2). Using incidence rates for the later period of 1978-1982, in all seven areas of the United States with such data, higher incidence rates were recorded in whites than in blacks with the excess ranging between 10% and 33% of the baseline black rate. Thus, there is a strong degree of consistency between the findings of higher breast cancer incidence rates in whites than in black members of the same community.

Incidence data are available from 15 regions of the world where a district can be separated into areas of urban or rural residence.

In all these 15 regions, covering the period 1973-1977, the incidence of breast cancer was found to be higher in the urban as opposed to the rural area, irrespective of whether the district lay in a high or low risk continent (Table 3).

The excess in incidence was approximately 50% ranging from (ignoring extreme values) an excess of 19% to 89%. Muir provide data for the period 1978-1982 from 11 regions. Again, in all regions the breast cancer incidence rate is consistently higher in urban as opposed to rural areas and (again ignoring extreme values) the excess ranges from 11% to 66% (Table 3).

Table 2. Age-standardised incidence rates per 100,000 for breast cancer among "blacks" and "whites" in areas of the United States (from Muir et al.)

	Whites	Blacks	Relative Risk
Alameda	78.4	68.4	1.15
Bay Area	87.0	66.4	1.31
Los Angeles	77.3	59.1	1.31
Connecticut	77.8	61.3	1.27
Atlanta	75.4	56.6	1.33
New Orleans	67.8	61.7	1.10
Detroit	74.9	63.4	1.18

Table 3. Breast cancer incidence in urban / rural populations

		Urban	Rural	Relative Risk
Japan	Fukuoka	15.8	12.1	1.31
	Miyagi	20.4	14.1	1.35
	Osaka	12.9	8.9	1.45
Czech	Slovakia	47.2	26.6	1.77
Finland		46.7	31.8	1.47
France	Bas-Rhin	55.5	54.0	1.03
	Doubs	73.7	39.0	1.89
Hungary	Szabolcs	27.6	18.9	1.46
Norway		55.0	44.8	1.23
Poland	Cieszyn	22.9	16.2	1.41
	Katowice	25.1	19.1	1.31
Spain	Zaragoza	46.1	19.8	2.33
Switzerland	Vaud	80.9	60.6	1.33
UK	North-Western	54.2	37.6	1.46
Australia	NSW	55.0	46.4	1.19

It seems clear that some aspects of urban living are associated with a 30-50% increase in breast cancer incidence over residence in rural areas of the same community.

Logan calculated cumulative rates of breast cancer according to broad socio-economic groups. His data show consistent evidence of an excess of breast cancer among the higher socio-economic groups when compared to the lowest groups. There is less evidence of this among single women. Members of the Church of Latter Day Saints (Mormons) in Utah have lower breast cancer incidence rates than would have been expected had either the rate among non-Mormons in the State, or the rates calculated in the Third National Cancer Survey (TNCS) been in force.

The Standardised Incidence Ratio of 82% in Mormons compared with TNCS was significantly reduced ($p<0.05$) while the comparative figure for non-Mormon women in Utah was increased (SIR=117).

Breast cancer has been shown to occur more frequently in Jews than in non-Jews, among Parsis as compared to Hindus, Moslems and Christians, and Old Order Amish, although no difference was found among Seventh Day Adventists and Hutterites.

A study among members of the Vegetarian Society of Great Britain revealed a higher proportional mortality for breast cancer than was expected according to the national rates. Detailed examination revealed that cases were of a higher socio-economic status and more likely to be unmarried than in general; this undoubtedly would lead to increased risk. Kinlen had earlier reported finding no difference in the breast cancer mortality rates among meat-eating and non-meat-eating nuns, although he noticed that neither group had lower mortality than the reference of all single women. This may explain observations of higher occurrence rates in nuns than have been documented consistently since Ramazzini.

Breast cancer has been consistently found to occur more frequently in women of higher socio-economic status as assessed by occupation or educational level or income. Socio-economic indicators by themselves are not the direct risk factor, but are strongly associated with other factors; for example Parsis tend to be more affluent than other members of the community in Western India and also tend to marry less frequently, at a later age and to have their first child later and to have fewer children. Studies of migrants have contributed significantly to recent hypotheses regarding breast cancer. The best studied migrants are those who left Japan for Hawaii or the West Coast of the United States. Studies of these migrants are consistent with an increase in breast cancer risk among second, and particularly among third, generation migrants. Boyle demonstrated extraordinarily high levels of breast cancer within the age range 40-65 in Japanese population groups within the United States. These data were interpreted in the following way: the older age groups were exclusively first generation and at increasingly younger ages the mixture becomes increasingly more second generation and subsequently third generation at the youngest ages. The high age-specific rates attained by Japanese migrants in the United States is surprising and the possibility that rates in migrants will overtake those in whites in years to come deserves close surveillance. Armstrong described the results for an analysis of cancer mortality in migrants to Australia compared to native-born Australians. Higher standardised rate ratios were found in women born in New Zealand, England and Wales, Scotland, Ireland and Germany where breast cancer mortality rates are higher than those recorded in Australia. In contrast, migrants from Greece, Italy and Poland, where lower rates of breast cancer are to be found, have lower breast cancer rates than native born Australians. When analysed by duration of residence, it is clear that as the duration of residence in Australia increases, so too the rate of breast cancer in these immigrant groups approaches that in native born Australians.

Summary of Descriptive Epidemiology

Different populations throughout the world experience different levels of breast cancer and these levels change with time in a regular manner. Within countries, breast cancer rates vary among racial groups, by socio-economic status, among different religious groups and by urban/rural residence; groups whose lifestyle differentiates them from other members of the same population. When migration takes place, groups of migrants tend to acquire the breast cancer pattern of their new home although it takes many years as in Australia, or generations as among Japanese arriving in the United States, for these changes to occur; this latter observation clearly indicates that it may be factors operating earlier in life which determine breast cancer risk. For reasons such as those presented above, it is believed that environmental factors rather than genetic factors are of paramount importance in the aetiology of this cancer; "environment" being defined in its broadest sense to include a wide range of factors such as dietary, social and cultural practices. The implication is, therefore, that breast cancer may be preventable and that there are practical prospects for breast cancer reduction. To identify and alter the factors which cause rates to be higher in urban as opposed to rural areas would reduce breast cancer by approximately 30 to 50 percent. Similarly, to identify the risk factors responsible for the excess in whites over blacks in the same community could reduce breast cancer by between 30% and 50%. Similar reductions are possible for identifying factors associated with being a member of the Church of Latter Day Saints (Mormons) and slightly lower reductions associated simply with socio-economic status. Identification and alteration of the relevant risk factors may render a portion of breast cancer avoidable.

Analytical Epidemiology

Given the recognised influence of ovarian function and hormone production on breast cancer growth and development, it is not surprising that much of the accumulated literature regarding the aetiology of breast cancer has focused on factors such as menarche, menopause and childbirth which are capable of altering the hormonal milieu in the breast. Normal breast epithelial cells respond markedly at puberty and during pregnancy, indicating sensitivity to the hormones and growth factors whose concentrations change at these times. Furthermore, it is natural to consider that factors such as oral contraceptive usage and hormone therapy for whatever reason, which can influence levels of hormone growth factors, might also influence breast epithelial cell division and hence increase or decrease the chances of cell transformation.

Pregnancy-Related Factors

There would appear to be an overall 50% increase in breast cancer risk in nulliparous as opposed to parous women. Ramazzini showed that nuns had an increased risk of breast cancer over other women and Rigoni-Stern calculated that the risk was increased by 5-fold. This association with nulliparity has been continually and consistently demonstrated using either zero parity or a surrogate measure "unmarried" as the variable of interest. It is also clear that the effect of parity is not simple and seems to depend strongly on how many births take place and at what age. It is also important to consider live births differently from miscarriages and abortions.

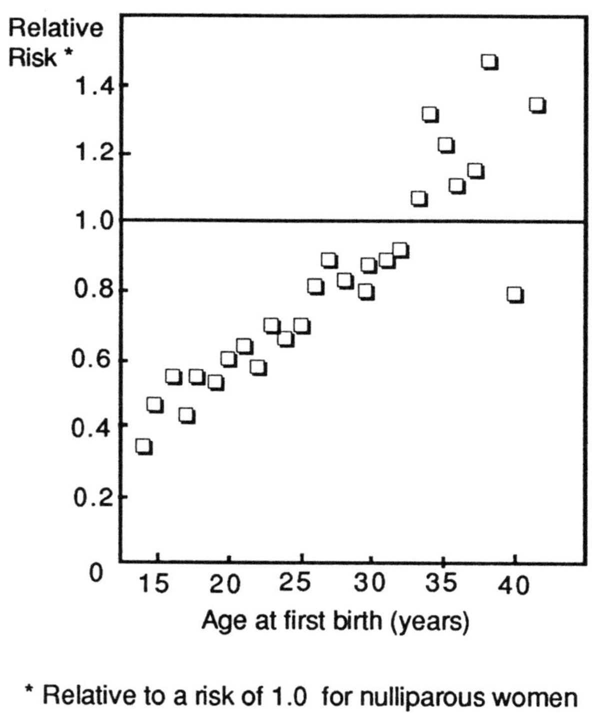

Fig. 5. Age at first birth and breast cancer risk: results from Seven Country International Study of MacMahon et al. (1970)

The international collaborative study conducted in seven centres at varying risk of breast cancer around the mid-1960s found the risk in parity 5+ to be between 40-60% that in nulliparous women. When the authors examined age at first birth, it was clear there was protection conferred by having birth at an early age and that the risk approached that of nulliparous women as age at first birth increased. It was also apparent that in women whose first birth occurred after the age of 35, there was an increased risk over nulliparous women. This is clearly demonstrated in Figure 5, taken from MacMahon, showing the effect of age at first birth by single years of age.

MacMahon also clearly showed that the effect of age at first birth remained after controlling for parity. The same study concluded that births after the first appeared to confer little or no further protection. Many of the earlier studies of breast cancer found risk to be increased with low parity although they could not adjust for the effects of other risk factors. Kvale, Heuch and Eide reported a cohort study from Norway which demonstrated a strong protective effect with increasing number of children from one to a group with 9+ parity: this result was independent of age at first birth.

There remains great conflict in the epidemiological literature about the independent contribution of age at first birth and parity to the risk of breast cancer.

Among 22 epidemiological studies on breast cancer published since 1970, 5 showed an association with age at first birth but not parity, 9 showed an association with both multiparity and age at first birth, 7 showed an association with parity but not age at first birth and 1 showed no significant association with both sets of reproductive factors. When all these studies are considered simultaneously, it would appear that breast cancer risk increases with increasing age at first birth and also that risk decreases with increasing parity, although the largest protective effects do not manifest themselves until parities of 4 or more.

Kvale and Heuch found an initial association between early age at first birth and breast cancer which was removed after adjustment for parity and age at last birth. After adjustment for parity, age at last birth showed a significant positive association with breast cancer risk at least in breast cancer cases diagnosed before the age of 70. These findings are essentially new and require to be confirmed in a variety of population groups, although there is already some support for their hypotheses published.

It is clear that the association between pregnancy-related events and breast cancer risk still requires clarification at some point. What is emerging from Trichopoulos and Kvale is the possibility that on top of the effects of parity and age at first birth there could well be an adverse effect associated with births occurring after the age of 35. It could be argued that there are two possible explanations to explain the apparent association between early age at first birth and the reduced risk of breast cancer; either a direct protective effect of an early first birth or of a confounding factor which reduces fertility and thereby delays pregnancy. Lilienfeld analysed data from two case-control studies and clearly showed that it is an early first birth and not reduced fertility which reduces the risk of breast cancer.

Many studies of breast cancer focused on breast feeding as a possible risk factor. After a large number of studies apparently demonstrated a protective effect, Thomas clearly showed the protective effect of breast feeding was confined to studies which could not control for parity. The possible association was discarded until the striking finding of a protective effect of breast feeding found in a study from New York State which revealed a negative association between duration of breast feeding and breast cancer risk in premenopausal women which was not found in post-menopausal women. Byers concluded that either breast feeding was truly protective or that some women who are unsuccessful at breast feeding are at an increased breast cancer risk, and they could not choose between these two hypotheses since cases reported more frequently than controls unsuccessful lactations due to "insufficient milk". Failure to lactate properly could be an indicator of some underlying hormonal imbalance which could possibly increase the risk of breast cancer. Skegg concluded that the recent evidence suggested that earlier theories about the protective effects of breast cancer could have been discarded prematurely.

Several studies showed an increased risk of breast cancer associated with miscarriages or spontaneous abortions while other studies have demonstrated no relationship. Pike reported a relative risk of 2.4 of breast cancer among young women (under age 33) who had a first trimester abortion (either spontaneous or induced) before their first full-term pregnancy. This is an important finding in view of the increasing numbers of abortions taking place prior to first full-term pregnancy in many countries and requires substantiating, because if the effect persists into later ages when breast cancer is commoner, it could bring about striking increases in incidence.

Factors Related to Menses

The reported association between age at menarche and breast cancer risk could best be described as weak, although there are suggestions that an early age at menarche increases breast cancer risk. While dispute about this association is to be found in case control studies, prospective studies from various countries such as Iceland, New York and the United States have all reported increased breast cancer risk with early menarche.

The association with a late age at natural menopause and an increased risk of breast cancer is more clearly defined. Breast cancer risk is perhaps doubled in late menopause compared with early menopause; setting the risk as 1.0 in the group with menopause at age 45-54, risks of 0.73 were found in the group who had menopause before age 45 and 1.48 in those who had menopause after age 55. Ewertz and Duffy reported the risk to be 1.67 among women who had a menopause after 55 as compared to those who had a menopause at ages before 45 (RR=1.0); the trend was highly significant.

There is also a strong body of evidence demonstrating the protective effect of artificial menopause on breast cancer risk and this protection is only conferred apparently when oophorectomy accompanies hysterectomy; hysterectomy along does not appear to alter the risk. Bilateral oophorectomy seems necessary to confer maximum risk reduction with the degree of protection less in women with unilateral oophorectomy or menopause induced by pelvic radiation. Trichopoulos, MacMahon and Cole reported that if oophorectomy was performed prior to age 35, the risk of breast cancer relative to women who experienced natural menopause between the ages 45-54 was 0.36.

Age at menarche and age at menopause are related to total life time years of menstrual activity and there is some evidence that this may be associated with breast cancer risk, although the difficulties of separating the three effects are apparent. There is conflicting evidence regarding an association between breast cancer risk and menstrual irregularity and length of menstrual cycles, and little evidence of an association with other features of menstrual activity such as pain during menstruation, duration of flow, amount of flow, and painful alterations to breasts during menstruation. In reviewing these facets of menstrual activity, Thomas concluded that they appear to be of little importance in the aetiology of breast cancer.

Oral Contraceptive Usage

The most obvious alteration to the hormonal status of women has been the widespread availability and use of oral contraceptives since the early 1960s. In recent years there have been many conflicting reports of the health effects of these preparations and much emotion still surrounds the issue. A recent comprehensive review by Prentice and Thomas provided a much needed and timely addition to the scientific debate. Taken together, the results of all the studies of oral contraceptive use and breast cancer risk have been generally reassuring although there is increasing evidence of a risk associated with use at an early age or before first-term birth, and that this risk is particularly elevated among women who developed breast cancer at a younger age. It must be remembered that observation time is at present about the maximum of 20 years and there could theoretically be a major effect which has not yet shown up due to latency. MacPherson, Coope and Vessey considered the theoretical effect of latency in a thoughtful manner and conclude that if oral contraceptives acted as a promoter in early stage carcinogenesis, the risk associated with oral contraceptive usage may not yet be observable. This situation, as with the possible downward trends in breast cancer discussed earlier, and which would conflict with the "oral contraceptive hypothesis", requires surveillance and continual investigation.

Non-Contraceptive Exogenous Oestrogens

Case-control studies of (non-contraceptive) exogenous oestrogens provide little clear indication of an increased risk when considered as a ever/never phenomenon. Some consistency becomes apparent, however, when the doses received are considered. Risk of breast cancer seems to increase with increasing "dose" of menopausal oestrogens. Similarly, studies of diethylstiboestrol (DES) show that breast cancer risk is highest in those who receive the highest dose. Two cohort studies of DES mothers estimate a risk of 2.0, although the risk associated with spontaneous abortions/miscarriage (for which DES was given) could account for a good proportion of this excess. Thomas cited case reports of breast cancer in two transvestite men who received large doses of oestrogens to induce breast development as additional evidence regarding the carcinogenic nature of oestrogen and there have been subsequent case reports of this phenomenon.

Benign Breast Disease

Women who have had fibrocystic breast disease are found to have a 2-3 fold increased risk of breast cancer which persists for up to 30 years after the fibrocystic disease has been diagnosed. In a large study of consecutive breast biopsies, it was demonstrated that the majority of women (70%) who underwent a biopsy for benign breast disease were not at an increased risk of cancer, and that the risk was increased by the presence of atypical hyperplasia with women having this feature with an approximate 4-fold increase in breast cancer risk over a general population.

Dietary Factors

Much of the evidence linking breast cancer risk to dietary parameters has been derived from correlational studies between breast cancer incidence and mortality with per capita intake of total fat and other nutrients in a variety of countries. Results from such ecological studies have provided statistically significant correlations between fat intake and the risk of breast cancer. Although such studies provide only a weak form of epidemiological evidence and generally there is a stronger correlation with gross national product, they have been influential in forming our understanding of the aetiology of breast cancer. Direct studies in women with and without breast cancer continue to offer the most relevant epidemiological evidence and will therefore form the basis of this section.

Obesity, Physical Activity and Energy Intake

There seems to be an increased risk of breast cancer among obese women, at least at postmenopausal ages, although not every study has been consistent in this finding. There also seems to be an association between obesity and an increased rate of occurrence after mastectomy. Obesity, related to the net balance of energy intake and energy expenditure, thus seems to have a central role in the aetiology of breast cancer, although the specific role is not yet clear. Physical activity, or some related consequence, has been shown to have a protective effect on the risk of breast cancer, even after adjustment for other confounding (risk) factors. However, studies such as those of Willett have failed to find the risk increased by reported total intake of energy.

Dietary Fat Intake

Results of direct studies on women with breast cancer provide conflicting evidence for an association between fat intake and the risk of breast cancer. The findings from some studies are so clear and internally consistent, however, that they cannot be ignored. Although few are statistically signficant, many of the case control studies of dietary fat are consistent with a small increase in the risk of breast cancer. On the other hand, prospective studies have to date provided absolutely no support to the dietary fat hypothesis, nor even to a possible association with meat intake. Although biologically plausible, there seems to be no consistent evidence from direct studies of women with breast cancer to support the association of risk of the disease with current fat intake or total energy intake or protein intake. The most powerful epidemiological study to date (in terms of the prospective design, methodology and sample size) - The Prospective Nurses's Health Study in the United States - reported no evidence of any increased risk associated with the intake of total fat, saturated fat, linoleic acid or cholesterol in either pre-menopausal or post-menopausal women. However, the possibility remains that dietary influences in early life, especially at puberty, are important determinants of breast cancer risk, influencing risk by affecting endocrine function.

The important issue of dietary intake and breast cancer risk needs urgent resolution. Though the situation with energy intake and fat intake remains unclear at present, findings of a protective effect associated with the consumption of vegetables require confirmation.

Alcohol Intake

Several recent studies have shown an association between alcohol consumption and an increased risk of female breast cancer with only a few of the published studies contradicting these findings. Evidence of an association is becoming stronger although the risks reported are generally small (around 1.5); the alcohol habit, however, is so widespread in Western countries that the possibility remains that it could account for a large proportion of breast cancer.
Although most studies have generally found associations between modest levels of alcohol intake and breast cancer risk, it is not yet clear that this association is causal. This literature has been summarised as suggesting a need for women to be recommended to moderate their alcohol consumption until the situation is clarified.

Reduction of Breast Cancer Risk through Dietary Modification

It is generally reported that obesity increases the risk of breast cancer, at least among postmenopausal women. It is a natural consequence to expect that aspects of nutrition, particularly energy intake, should have an influential role in the aetiology of breast cancer. To date there is no clear evidence that either energy intake or the dietary sources of energy (fat, protein and carbohydrates) are important in the aetiology of breast cancer in women. These findings, particularly related to dietary fat intake, are in direct conflict with the results of ecological studies and animal experiments. There seems to be some indication of a protective effect associated with increased consumption of fresh vegetables and evidence of a possible association between the risk of breast cancer and alcohol intake. To advise women to reduce obesity, brought about by a reduction in energy intake from all sources, an increase in consumption of fresh vegetables and fruits, and moderation of alcohol intake, would be sound advice. Such dietary prudence would also be undoubtedly beneficial in reducing the risk of other common diseases, even if it did not turn out to have a great effect on reducing the risk of breast cancer.

Family History of Breast Cancer

It is almost uniformly reported that women with a first degree relative with breast cancer are at an increased risk of developing breast cancer themselves. This risk is most strongly influenced by the mother, since the risk is much higher in women with a mother and sister affected than in women with a sister alone. The risk seems to be particularly concentrated among women whose mother develops breast cancer at a premenopausal age. Horm and Thompson report a case-control study of contralateral breast cancer. A family history of breast cancer in any first or second degree relative was associated with a 2.8 fold increased risk of developing a contralateral breast cancer.

Ionising Radiation

Radiation to the breast in high doses has been shown to increase the risk of breast cancer, whether the radiation was from nuclear explosion, from treatment of acute post partum mastitis, women who received fluoroscopy or who are radiated for tinea capititis. Exposure of the breasts to radiation at ages 10-19 is associated with a particularly high risk, with the greatest risk associated with perimenarchial exposure. This suggests that breast tissue is particularly vulnerable at this time, because either the breasts are developing rapidly or because most women have not yet given birth.

Other Breast Cancer Risk Factors

A number of other risk factors have been shown by one or more studies to be involved in the aetiology of breast cancer. These include factors such as cigarette smoking, primary biliary cirrhosis, use of reserpine and certain hair dyes. These have been reviewed recently.

Diagnosis and Staging

Diagnostic Evaluation

The evaluation of the patient should begin with a careful history and physical examination. Visual examination of the patient sitting with the arms raised over the head may disclose evidence of a breast lump or skin alteration. Palpation may discover a breast mass, enlarged nodes and otherwise unapparent skin retraction may be provoked (pushing a breast lump towards the chest wall with the patient standing and leaning forward may be useful). Gentle pressure of the areola may be needed to evidence non-spontaneous nipple discharge.

Clinical findings which may be related to the local effects of the cancer include lump, nipple bloody discharge, nipple deviation or retraction, skin dimpling, oedema, infiltration or ulceration and enlarged axillary nodes. Development of a breast lump is the most common symptom, although of course it is quite nonspecific being possibly ascribed to many benign conditions. Bloody nipple discharge is a much more specific symptom although at least half of the cases are due to benign intraductal papillomas. Other types of discharge (watery, serous, milky, purulent) are only occasionally associated with cancer. Nipple deviation or retraction are not frequent symptoms of cancer and are often associated with grossly evident tumour. Nipple retraction due to retroareolar fibrosis may be found in elderly patients and may be a misleading sign when unilateral. Skin alteration is probably the most specific sign of cancer. It usually involves the skin overlying a palpable mass but may be occasionally an isolated sign. Infiltration and ulceration are highly specific and predictive of cancer. Oedema and dimpling are less specific, being possibly due to acute or chronic inflammatory disease, respectively. Enlarged axillary nodes are infrequently reported by the patient although they may be detected on physical examination. The presence of palpable axillary nodes is a very nonspecific symptom being often present, even bilaterally, in most women undergoing physical examination. Only enlarged nodes over 2 cm in diameter, or nodes fixed to surrounding structures are really worth regarding as suspicious.

The sensitivity of physical examination is greatly affected by tumour size as small tumours may be missed, especially in large breasts. Approximately 30% of tumours under 2 cm and the majority of tumours under 1 cm in diameter will be missed or misdiagnosed as benign by physical examination.

Thus, physical examination, while being cheap and simple, is neither specific nor sensitive for early breast cancer. As a general rule, physical examination should not be used alone and any abnormality should undergo further diagnostic work up. Moreover, a negative finding on physical examination should not be completely reassuring.

Mammography (conventional film technique or xeromammography are equivalent) is no doubt the most accurate test for breast cancer diagnosis. Breast cancers may be detectable even as small as 3-4 mm in diameter and over 85% of tumours smaller than 2 cm will be correctly diagnosed. Age is the major factor affecting the accuracy of mammography as the young breast is radiologically dense and may mask the presence of cancer. Still, mammography may reveal cancer even in a dense juvenile breast, especially if calcifications are present. Thus, mammography should be performed at any age even when only a minimal suspicion of cancer is present.

Cytology is the third fundamental test for breast cancer diagnosis. Cytologic examination of nipple discharge or of cyst fluid is advised only when blood is present. Non bloody discharge or cyst fluid are so rarely associated with cancer that their routine examination is not cost effective. Fine needle aspira-

tion cytology of all palpable masses of even minimal clinical suspicion (and of non-palpable lesions with proper stereotaxic or ultrasound-guided techniques) is mandatory. The technique is simple, cheap and safe and the risk of tumour dissemination is irrelevant. Inadequate sampling may be a problem but it can be easily ruled out by proper training of the operators. The diagnostic accuracy of cytology is heavily dependent on the expertise of the cytopathologist. Cytology is the most specific test presently available. The probability of cancer in the presence of a positive (cancer cells) cytologic report is over 99% and, especially when associated to plain evidence of cancer on physical examination and mammography, the risk of false positive reports is practically zero and peroperative frozen biopsy may be safely bypassed. The sensitivity for cancer is reported to be around 90%. A widespread use of fine needle aspiration cytology of any palpable solid mass may lead to correct identification of otherwise misdiagnosed cancer and treatment delay can thus be avoided.
Physical examination, mammography and cytology represent the fundamental tests for breast cancer detection and should be available in all breast clinics. Their combined use allows the highest accuracy and a further improvement by adding other presently available tests is unlikely.
Other techniques have been proposed for the diagnosis of breast cancer. Sonography is no doubt the first worth mentioning. It has the highest accuracy in differentiating cystic from solid lesions but this advantage is obviously largely lost by the widely used cheaper practice of aspiration of palpable masses which achieves diagnosis and treatment at the same time for cystic lesions. Sonography may be of help in the diagnostic work up of palpable solid masses in very dense juvenile breast as the test accuracy is not affected at younger ages as mammography is. Transillumination (including the recently developed spectroscopy employing infrared emission) is of limited advantage, being much less specific than mammography (most lesions appear just as shadows and no reliable differential diagnosis is possible). Thermography (infrared or contact technique are almost equivalent as far as the diagnostic information is considered) is increasingly abandoned by most centres due to its poor sensitivity, especially for smaller tumours. CT or MRI have no role in the current practice of primary breast cancer diagnosis.

Screening

Breast cancer is a major health problem due to its frequency and lethal effect.
Primary prevention is almost impossible as aetiologic factors are unclear and allow no practical preventive measures. Secondary prevention, by screening for asymptomatic, early stage breast cancer, has long been an attractive idea. Unfortunately, no suitable risk factor is presently available to select women to screening, apart from age, and screening would involve a large proportion of the female population. Several screening experiences have been carried out since the first controlled study which was started almost 20 years ago. All the studies thus far reporting mortality data confirm that screening has a significant impact on breast cancer mortality. Unfortunately, these studies are not homogeneous in design and involve relatively small populations.
Thus, further analysis of mortality results and of the optimal screening features is quite complicated. Breast cancer mortality is reduced by screening but the extent of this reduction seems to be age dependent. A significant reduction of mortality in women aged over 49 years has been reported in all studies whereas in women aged 40-49 the impact on breast cancer mortality was absent or not statistically significant. Mammography was of course the screening test of choice as it was the only one allowing preclinical detection. Physical examination was employed in addition to mammography in two studies which were not specifically designed to answer the question of the independent effectiveness of each technique.
Mammography seems to have the major role in mortality reduction, especially as modern mammography showed a dramatic improvement in quality in the 1970s, but a possible impact of physical examination on mortality reduction cannot be excluded, especially at younger ages when mammography is less

Evidence on breast cancer mortality reduction by screening

Study	Tests	Frequency (years)	Mortality reduction age 40-49	age > 49
Randomized studies (invited vs. controls)				
H.I.P.*	M + PE	1	21 % **	23 %
Sweden	M	2-3	none	39 %
Malmoe	M	2	no data	20%**
UK trial	M + (PE)	2 (1)	no data	46%
Case-control studies (responders vs. non responders)				
Florence	M	2.5	24 % **	62 %
Utrecht	M + PE	1-2	no data	70 %
Nijmegen	M	2	none	51 %

* 14 year evaluation ** Statistically not significant , M = mammography, P = physical examination

sensitive. The optimal rescreening interval is still to be assessed. Breast cancer mortality has been significantly reduced with quite different rescreening intervals, ranging from 1 to 3 years.

In conclusion, convincing evidence is available supporting the fact that screening may reduce breast cancer mortality. Large-scale screening in asymptomatic women can now be advocated as a public health policy. Screening programmes on a national basis are going to be implemented in Northern Europe. The optimal screening features are controversial and need further investigation before being definitively assessed. Different screening protocols are likely to be almost equally effective though they may greatly differ as far as organisation and costs are concerned. Screening healthy women aged 50 to 70 with mammography alone every two years seems a reasonable option which is likely to be cost effective and feasible even on a national scale. Considering the radiation dose presently delivered by modern mammography, the risk of radioinduced cancer is irrelevant and by far outweighed by screening benefits.

Staging

Staging is aimed at defining the extent of the disease in order to assess proper treatment. Axillary nodes are the most common site of locoregional diffusion and their clinical status is always to be investigated. Unfortunately, physical examination is not reliable as about one third of clinically suspected nodes will show no histological involvement which will be otherwise present in about one third of clinically negative axillas. The evidence of large nodes fixed to surrounding structures is a high predictive sign of nodal involvement but is quite infrequent (less than 1% of cases). In the large majority of cases, surgical excision of axillary nodes is the current procedure and nodal status is pathologically assessed. Supraclavicular and internal mammary node involvement is quite infrequent at the time of first diagnosis and usually associated with advanced, often inoperable primary tumours. Physical examination and fine needle aspiration cytology are the diagnostic methods of choice. Breast cancer infrequently presents with evidence of distant metastases at first diagnosis. Symptoms from distant spread usually occur after primary treatment and their presence as the only symptom at initial diagnosis is definitely rare. Physical examination may reveal bone tenderness, irregular hepatomegaly, neurological disorders or soft tissue nodules. In the latter event, fine needle aspiration cytology may be of great help in differential diagnosis. Bone scintigraphy provides a valuable assessment of the whole skeleton. False positives are common with hot spots of the scan due to degenerative conditions or old trauma especially at older ages. Further work up of hot spots should be carried out by standard X-ray or tomography to exclude other causes. False negatives are infrequent but if clinical suspicion of bone metastases is present radiological studies are needed.

Standard two-views chest X-ray is the test of choice for the diagnosis of intrathoracic metastases to lung, pleura or mediastinum. Diagnostic work up of questionable cases is usually performed by conventional or computerised tomography. In the presence of pleural effusion cytologic examination of aspirated fluid is mandatory. Liver and brain metastases are infrequently reported as first site of recurrence. Hepatic ultrasound has been shown to be more sensitive than isotope scans and as good as CT scanning. CT scanning of the brain is no doubt more sensitive than isotope scan. Blood tests (serum alkaline phosphatase, CEA, urinary hydroxyproline etc.) may be altered in the presence of distant metastases but the elevation of circulating markers is usually strictly related to the extent of the tumour burden. Blood tests are usually altered in the late course of the disease, that is, when symptomatic metastases are already known. The probability that asymptomatic and subclinical metastases are detected in this way is quite limited and by far outweighed by the risk of false positivity. The evidence of distant spread at initial diagnosis greatly influences the decision on the optimal treatment option including the need for radical surgery. Thus, a careful search for distant metastases, even subclinical, is often advocated in asymptomatic patients. Chest X-ray and bone scan are usually employed for this purpose. However, the detection rate of asymptomatic and subclinical metastases is very small, usually less than 2%, whereas at least 50% of operable patients actually have and will have developed distant metastases after ten years since first treatment. The sensitivity of preoperative staging for subclinical metastases is thus very low. Moreover, false positives are expected which may cause treatment delay because of the necessary diagnostic work up, and possibly undertreatment in those cases in which false positives are not ruled out and radical surgery is not performed. On the other hand a bad treatment decision due to insufficient staging procedures may be a heavy burden on a few patients and the availability of baseline documentation at the start of treatment may also be of some use. In conclusion, the policy of preoperative staging for the detection of subclinical and asymptomatic distant metastases has its pros and cons. It can be suggested that one might currently adopt it though being aware of its limited sensitivity and high costs.

Follow up

Periodic follow up of breast cancer patients after primary treatment is a common practice. Physical examination and mammography are commonly performed in order to detect locoregional recurrences (axillary, supraclavicular or internal mammary) or contralateral primary cancer. Cure is possible, especially as regards contralateral cancer and axillary recurrences, when early detection is achieved, and it is most likely that such a follow up policy may have a favourable though limited impact on prognosis. Symptoms and signs of distant metastases should be carefully looked for at periodic physical examination. As for many other solid tumours, a large variety of symptoms may be ascribed to disseminated disease. Pain due to bony metastases may be present. The bones most frequently involved are the spine, pelvis, femur, ribs and skull although any bone may be affected. Pain from hepatomegaly, dyspnoea or thoracic pain from massive lung metastases or pleural dissemination and systemic effects of breast cancer (anorexia, weakness, weight loss) are usually late symptoms and an infrequent pattern of first metastatic recurrence. Instrumental tests in search of subclinical metastases are often performed at periodic follow up examinations. Although early detection of subclinical metastases is possible there is no clinical evidence that a better prognosis is achieved when treatment of metastatic disease is applied in the subclinical phase rather than after the onset of symptoms. Patients with early detected asymptomatic metastases usually have a longer survival than symptomatic patients but this difference might be entirely ascribed to the lead time effect of diagnostic anticipation, survival being measured from the date of metastasis detection.

Retrospective studies comparing asymptomatic to symptomatic metastatic patients tend to deny any difference in survival from the time of primary treatment. Prospective randomised studies are ongoing which probably will definitely answer the question of the cost effectiveness of periodic performance of instrumental tests to detect subclinical metastases. Presently this policy seems questionable as benefits are uncertain and the economic and psychological costs are high.

Pathology

Malignant epithelial tumours of the breast must first be divided into non-infiltrating and infiltrating carcinomas.

Non-Invasive Carcinoma

Lobular carcinoma in situ (LCIS) is generally revealed as an incidental histological finding on the occasion of a breast biopsy performed for a benign lesion. Cancer cells are crowded into a lobular structure without any signs of invasion. It is often multicentric and bilateral and it represents a "risk factor" of some significance. Patients who have been found to have LCIS foci in their breast are exposed to a risk of subsequent invasive breast carcinoma 5 to 10 times higher than that of the general population.

Ductal carcinoma in situ (DCIS) is a type of carcinoma being diagnosed more and more frequently as a result of the extensive use of mammography which can pick up non-palpable lesions through the appearance of microcalcifications. DCIS can be divided into three main pathological types: microfocal (<0,5 cm. in diameter), diffuse and tumour-forming. Histologically, the most common forms are the papillary and the solid types, whilst the cribriform type is less frequent. When the central part of the lumen undergoes a necrotic process the pattern is defined as comedo-like. DCIS is often multicentric (20% of the cases) and sometimes bilateral (5-10%). The type of spread is mainly intraductal, so that it may grow silently for a long time, without any clinical signs, filling the ducts of portions of the mammary gland. It may reach the nipple and grow in the epidermis of the areolar and periareolar skin: in this case it is defined as Paget's disease.

In principle, the cell proliferation being non-infiltrating, there is no possibility of spread to the regional lymph nodes. The exceptional cases of axillary metastases described (2%) are probably due to inadequate sampling of the primary tumour by the pathologists who, thereby, may have overlooked small areas of invasion.

Invasive Carcinoma

Invasive ductal carcinoma (IDC) is the most common type of breast cancer (70% of the total), the pathological appearance of which is usually a hard, stellate nodule with a white-grey surface. Histology may be very different from one case to another. In some cases of IDC, small DCIS foci may be discovered at the periphery of the mass. When the presence of DCIS is extensive, the case is defined as "invasive ductal carcinoma with a predominant intraductal component". The recognition of this entity is important, as it is one of the most important factors in the risk of recurrence in conservative surgery.

The peritumoral spread may occur through invasion of blood and lymphatic vessels by tumour emboli. When this occurs the prognosis is worse. Multifocality (multiple foci close to each other around the primary tumour) is uncommon (3%), whilst multicentricity (multiple foci distant from each other) is found in some 10% of cases

Invasive lobular carcinoma (ILC) is also a frequent type (10-15% of the total) characterised histologically by a single-file, linear cellular arrangement, although other variants have been described (trabecular, alveolar, tubular). In ILC the peritumoral intravascular invasion is rare. The pattern of spread and the prognosis of ILC is not different from those of IDC.

In some 5-10% of the cases the ILC pattern is mixed with that of IDC.

Uncommon types with favourable prognoses are: medullary carcinoma (4%) which is

roughly similar in appearance to fibroadenoma, mucinous carcinoma (2%), the main component of which is a colloid substance (the cellularity may be less than 10% of the tumour mass), papillary carcinoma (1%) which may produce nipple discharge, tubular carcinoma (1%), often accompanied by a high degree of fibrosis, adenoid cystic carcinoma, similar to that arising in the salivary glands, by mucoepidermoid carcinomas.
All these pathological entities form a special group of breast tumours which represent 8-10% of the total number of cases, generally with an excellent prognosis.
Inflammatory carcinoma represents 1-2% of all breast cancers and is histologically characterised by an extensive intralymphatic spread around the tumour with frequent invasion of the lymphatics of the dermis (which produces the classic clinical sign "peau d'orange").

Breast Sarcomas

This is a very rare type of breast pathology, consisting mainly of: fibrosarcomas (with good prognosis) and angiosarcomas (with poor prognosis). Primary malignant lymphomas (Hodgkin's and non-Hodgkin's) are also rare.

Philloid Tumours

This singular type of breast tumour, which is not uncommon, derives its original name from its foliated structure and is of particular importance for its tendency to recur locally. In fact, contrary to fibroadenoma, it is not encapsulated and for radical excision a wide margin of healthy tissue around the mass must be removed with the tumour. Philloid tumours are divided into a benign form (60%), a potentially malignant one (20%), and a malignant form (20%). The main criterion for classification is the mitotic index, together with the degree of cellularity and atypia. The malignant variant is locally very aggressive, with not uncommon blood-borne distant spread (25%) to lungs and liver. Lymphatic dissemination does not occur as a rule and axillary nodes are never involved.

Treatment: General Strategy

The approach to breast cancer treatment must follow a logical sequence in order to achieve a rational management of the disease. Such action will have the objective of acquiring information regarding the nature and the extent of the disease in order to be able to direct the surgical, radiological and medical therapies in the most effective way.

The five major steps in this process are :
1) diagnosis;
2) staging;
3) treatment of primary carcinoma and regional nodes;
4) post-surgical evaluation;
5) treatment of occult metastases.

The correct diagnosis of a breast carcinoma is obviously a preliminary requirement for conducting an appropriate treatment plan. Once the clinical and mammographic findings give rise to a suspicion of carcinoma, generally, a fine-needle biopsy will provide final evidence of malignancy. In some cases, however, a histological examination is required, and a small incisional biopsy or a more extensive excisional biopsy is called for. Today, a treatment plan is not drawn up if a complete unequivocal biopsy is not available. The procedure has led to intraoperative diagnosis made on frozen section examination becoming quite exceptional.
Once the diagnosis is made, the clinical extent of the disease is evaluated: the regional nodes are carefully examined, as well as the distant organs which are the more common sites of metastases (lung, liver, skeleton).
If no distant metastases are found, the type of treatment of the primary tumour is decided upon. It may be limited to a breast quadrantectomy, or to a resection of the breast in the case of a small tumour, or it may involve a total mastectomy in the case of a large tumour. Generally, the axillary nodes are also removed. If surgery is limited to a part of the breast, radiotherapy on the remaining portion is always indicated.
Following surgery, a careful record is made of the pathological evaluation of the primary carcinoma (including the peritumoral lymphatic invasion), the presence and the number of axillary nodes involved and the biological characteristics of the tumour (presence and quantity of hormonal receptors, degree of proliferation, ploidy, oncogene amplification etc.) (Fig. 6,7).
These findings constitute the main guide to deciding on the possible treatment of occult metastases. As we do not know whether distant metastases are present in a latent, clinically undetectable form, the decision to perform this treatment or not (which is defined adjuvant treatment) is made according to the probability that metastases are effectively present. A careful assessment of all these factors, to which a score is given, will put the patient either in a group at high risk of recurrence, in which case adjuvant treatment (chemotherapeutic or endocrine) is proposed, or in a group at low risk of recurrence, where there will be no need for adjuvant treatment. More recently, it has been proposed that all women affected by an invasive breast carcinoma should receive "some kind" of adjuvant medical treatment after surgery. If this line should become the rule in the future, the factors determining the adjuvant treatment to be applied should no longer be the prognostic index, but the expected response of the cancer cells to the various drugs and hormones.

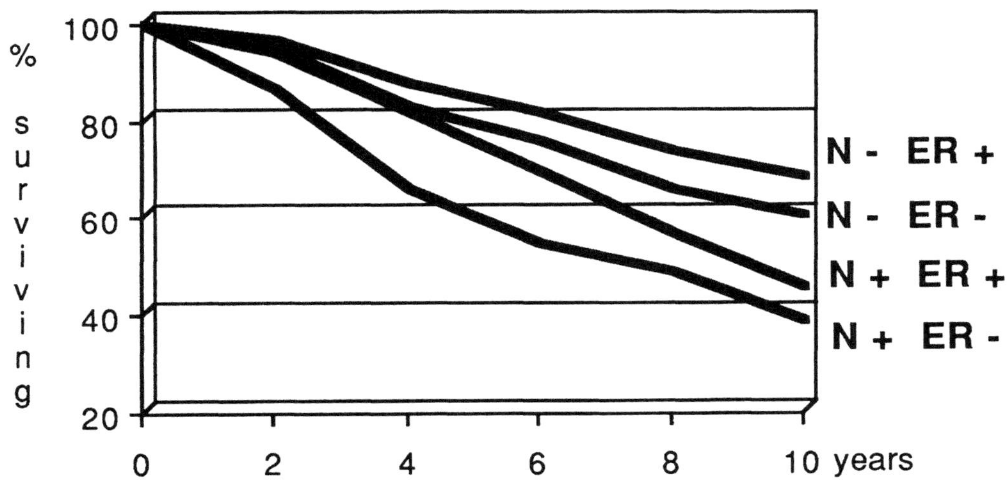

Fig. 6. Survival of breast cancer according to nodal status and oestrogen receptors

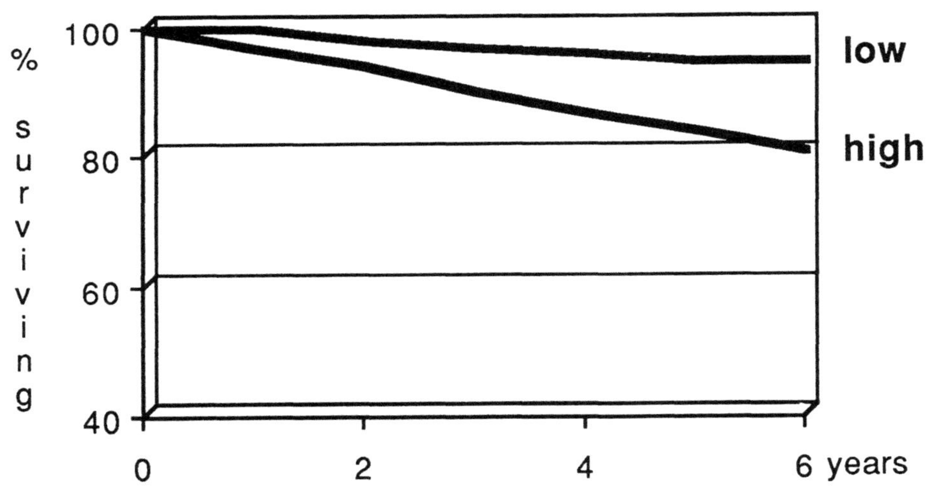

Fig. 7. Survival of node-negative breast cancer according to thymidine labelling index

Surgery

One hundred years ago W.S. Halsted opened up a new era in breast cancer treatment, introducing the "radical mastectomy". The principle of Halsted was that a rigourous, accurate surgical technique which would remove the breast "en bloc" with the pectoralis muscles and the axillary nodes would cure a considerable number of patients.
The need to remove the intermediate tissues from the primary breast tumour to the axillary nodes was based on the assumption that the spread of breast cancer cells would occur through the lymphatic vessels, with a process defined as "permeation", the cancer cell thereby "filling" all the major lymphatic channels departing from the breast. As some lymphatic ducts cross the pectoralis muscles their removal appeared consistent with these principles.
However, before the middle of this century, it was shown that the spread to the axillary nodes occurs through an "embolic" mechanism and not through the "permeation" process, undermining the basis for the "en bloc" operation. During these same years, new techniques were introduced which spared the major pectoralis muscle and which showed the same rates of survival.
After the Second World War, a group of surgeons, first in Europe and later in the USA, considered it necessary nonetheless to investigate the role of the internal mammary nodes in breast cancer treatment. If the removal of axillary nodes was considered a necessary component of the surgical treatment, they asked themselves, why should not the removal of the internal mammary nodes be considered equally important.
The extended radical mastectomy with dissection of the internal mammary node chain became rather popular for a certain number of years, but was later abandoned when an extensive clinical trial showed that long-term survival after extended mastectomy was not better than after the classic Halsted mastectomy (Fig. 8,9).
More recently, a number of clinical trials showed that mastectomy may be replaced by a lesser operation, such as the quadrantectomy, or lumpectomy (followed by RT), for tumours of small dimensions (Fig. 10).

At present, the suggested policy for breast cancer treatment may be summarised as follows:

❑ Lobular carcinoma in situ (LCIS). Simple careful follow up, with periodical mammography. In the case of multiple LCIS a subcutaneous mastectomy (plus immediate prosthetic replacement) may be considered.

❑ Ductal carcinoma in situ (DCIS). The indications may be total mastectomy, for extensive cases, subcutaneous mastectomy for less extensive tumours and breast resection or quadrantectomy (plus radiotherapy) for very circumscribed DCIS. No axillary dissection.

❑ Invasive carcinoma of less than 2-3 cm. The suggested surgical procedure is now the quadrantectomy followed by RT, with simultaneous axillary dissection. A simple local excision (lumpectomy - tumorectomy) may also be performed, although a higher rate of local recurrences may be expected. In the case of patients with very small breasts a total mastectomy with axillary dissection and immediate breast reconstruction may be preferable.

❑ Invasive carcinoma of more than 2-3 cm. The most widely used type of surgery is the total mastectomy and axillary dissection with or without immediate reconstruction.

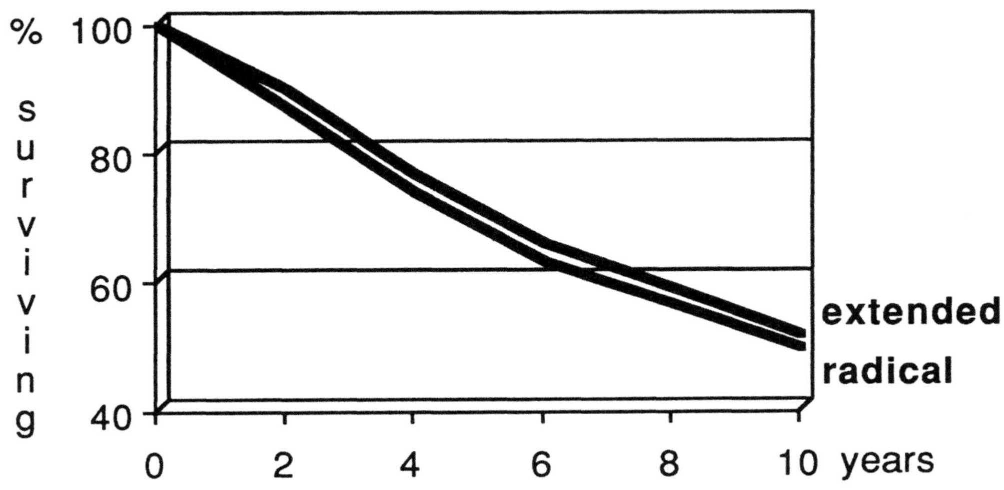

Fig. 8. Breast cancer survival: Halsted radical mastectomy versus extended mastectomy

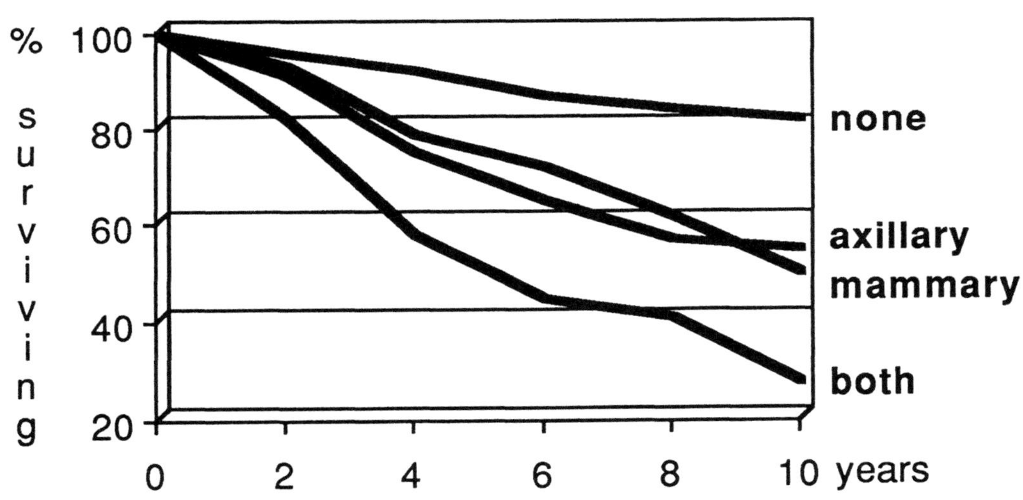

Fig. 9. Breast cancer survival by site of node metastases: patients without node metastases, with axillary node metastases only, with internal mammary node metastases only, and with both sites involved

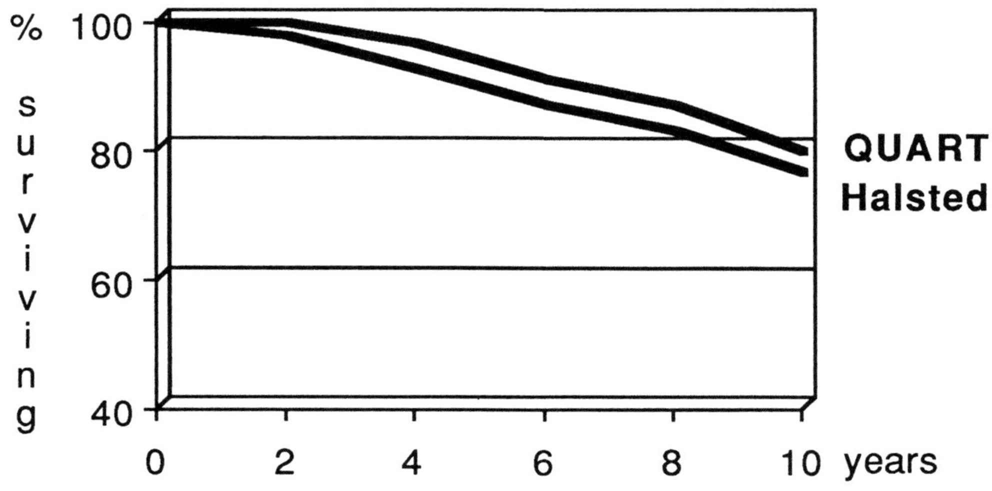

Fig. 10. Breast cancer survival: quadrantectomy versus Halsted (Milan Trial I)

❑ Very large carcinomas, fixed to the pectoralis muscle, with extensive axillary invasion may be treated (often after preoperative chemotherapy) with Halsted mastectomy.

❑ Inflammatory carcinoma. This aggressive type of carcinoma is generally treated with chemotherapy with or without radiotherapy. However, in cases showing a good regression of the primary tumour a Halsted mastectomy may be considered.

Reconstruction of the breast after mastectomy is more and more requested by women. Modern reconstructive techniques, together with the fact that the present-day surgical procedure generally preserves the major pectoralis muscle, provide good cosmetic results with relatively simple surgery. Reconstruction after an extensive Halsted mastectomy is more complicated, but satisfactory results may be obtained with the employment of musculo-cutaneous flaps, taken from the major thoraco-dorsal muscle and from the rectus abdominis muscle.

lumpectomy

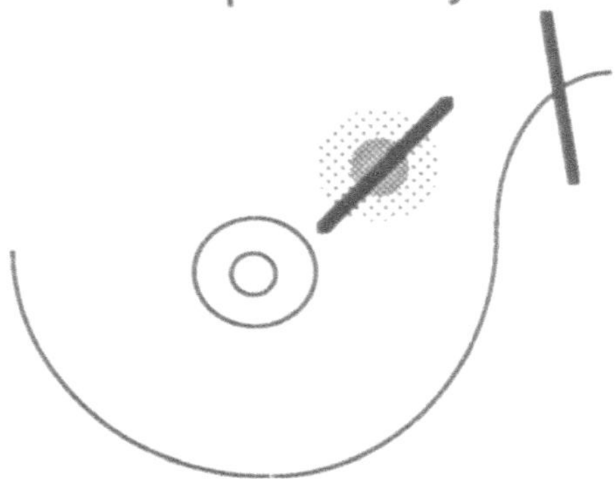

Removal of the primary carcinoma with a narrow margin of normal tissue.
The axillary dissection may be performed with a separate incision.

quadrantectomy

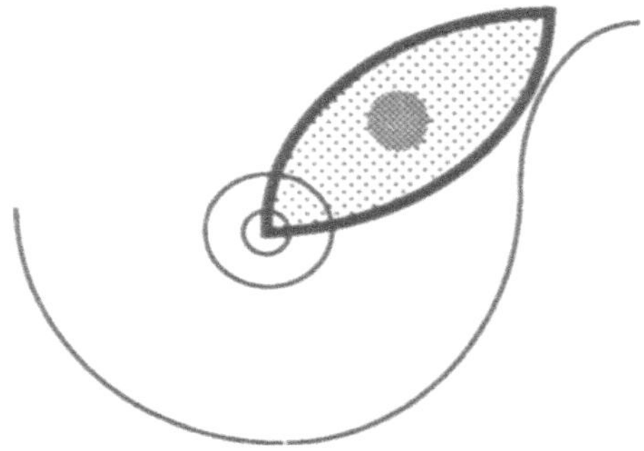

Removal of the quadrant harbouring the primary carcinoma with the overlying skin.
The axillary dissection may be performed in continuity (upper external quadrant) or with a separate incision.

total mastectomy

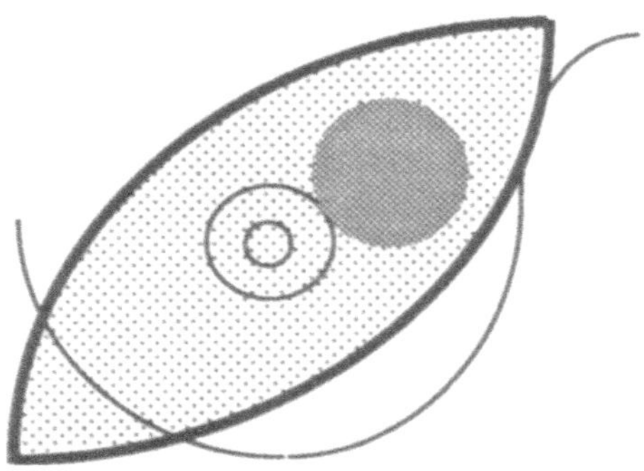

Removal of the whole breast together with the axillary nodes, sparing the pectoralis muscles.

Halsted mastectomy

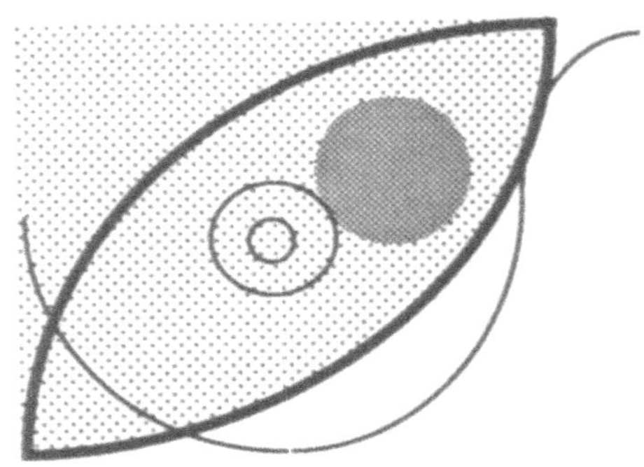

Removal of the whole breast together with the axillary nodes and both pectoralis muscles.

Radiotherapy

In recent decades, the concept has been developed that a breast cancer does not always require a mastectomy any more.
The aim of breast conserving treatment is to provide a therapy which achieves the same results as to a final cure of the patient, whilst reaching the highest possible percentage of patients, enabling them to keep their treated breast in a cosmetically satisfactory condition. Therefore, a careful balance has to be pursued between local control and treatment sequelae. Local recurrences have to be avoided as they are a potential source of secondary metastases, as they usually require rescue mastectomy, defeating the aim of the conserving therapy, and, finally, as they constitute an important psychological burden for the patients.
After very limited resections of the tumour, relapses develop in 25% of the patients. With the addition of postoperative radiotherapy to the breast this incidence of recurrence can be reduced to 5%-10%.
The study of the best balance between the extent of the surgical resection and the radiation dose level applied, as to their effect on the cosmetic outcome and local control is still ongoing. The initial approach of exclusive radiotherapy has been abandoned, as the doses necessary for controlling palpable disease induce too much late fibrosis.
While some centres carry out wide excisions (up to quadrantectomy), many others use a more limited surgery (tumorectomy with a safety margin of 1-2 cm) and moderately high radiation doses (60-65 Gy).
It is important to be well aware that, as is often the case, more limited treatments are technically much more complex than ablative treatments. This relates as well to the selection of patients suitable for such a procedure, as to the surgical procedure and the irradiation technique.
The radiation doses presently prescribed are close to the tolerance and it is therefore important to be able to irradiate the breast to as homogeneous a dose as possible.
The breast, when receiving a dose higher than prescribed, will develop sequelae which seriously hamper the cosmetic result. This is especially important as this is a patient population of which a large part will survive for very long periods after radiotherapy.
Also the problem of patient selection is very critical and requires a degree of sophistication on the part of the team of treating doctors. The indication for mastectomy was easy to make, only the inoperable cases having to be selected. The definition of the limits of breast conserving therapy is much more difficult.
In summary, breast conserving procedures are feasible and beneficial for a large group of patients. The selection of the patient group for which it must be applied, is critical and requires more experience and know-how than was the case for ablative procedures. The technique of irradiation, essential for obtaining good results, is also amongst the most difficult of radiotherapy techniques and requires a good infrastructure and wide experience.

Postoperative Irradiation of Breast Cancer

In earlier times, all patients with breast cancer were considered eligible for mastectomy. This also included patient groups which carried a very high incidence of local recurrence, such as tumours with signs of diffuse infiltration (e.g., mastitis, skin nodules at a distance) and patients with inoperable regional nodes. These patient groups led to high overall incidences of local relapses after mastectomy, which in turn resulted in the systematic postoperative irradiation of all patients.

A more critical selection of patients for mastectomy has led to local recurrence rates of less than five percent, rendering post-operative radiotherapy largely unnecessary.
The main parameters considered for such indications are very large tumours and non-radical resection margins.

Irradiation of Inoperable Breast Cancer

Patients for whom mastectomy is considered inadequate are now treated with radiotherapy. While many of these rapidly develop distant metastases, a sizable group of them survives for a fairly long period.
Good, long-term, local control is therefore mandatory for these patients. Carefully planned radiotherapy to high doses over the breast and the regional nodes is necessary in these patients.

Radiotherapy for Lymph Node Areas in Breast Cancer

The lymph node bearing areas in breast cancer are the axillary chain, which without any clear limit extends into the subclavian chain, and also the parasternal lymph nodes. Only the axillary chain is accessible for surgery. This is done, also for diagnostic purposes, in the course of curatively intended procedures, in clinically localised (breast and axillary nodes) breast cancer, since the axillary lymph node status is the best prognosticator for relapse and survival and is used often as the determining factor for adjuvant systemic therapy.
It has been common practice in the past to irradiate the lymph node areas as an adjunctive treatment to local surgery.
A benefit in terms of survival is not proven.
In a large number of studies no benefit has been shown, in a few others the small benefit seen was mainly in patients with central or medial origin of the tumour.
A benefit in terms of locoregional tumour control however is unquestionable: the recurrence rate in the lymph node areas is much lower in irradiated patients and there is even a clear influence of the radiation dose that is used (optimally 45-50 Gy). This benefit is mainly seen in patients at high risk for locoregional relapse (extensive axillary invasion, large primary tumours).
The large majority of patients with tumour in the lymph nodes will already have distant (subclinical) metastases.
Eradication of the tumour in the lymph nodes will not improve the survival in these patients. The group of patients with lymph node metastases but without distant metastases, is very small and it will be extremely difficult to find a beneficial effect on survival in studies comprising all patients. Furthermore, many of such irradiations in the past have been done with a radiation technology which is unacceptable today. While inadequate irradiation can reduce the incidence of relapses or delay their appearance, cure requires the inclusion of all existing tumour deposits to a sufficiently high dose for which the technique of irradiation is essential.
When radiotherapy is postponed to the time of regional recurrence, only half of the recurrences can be controlled, leaving these patients with substantial morbidity (arm oedema, nerve palsy, ulcers).
Patients with important invasion in the axillary lymph nodes, with central or medial tumour sites in the breast or with large tumours, may benefit from lymph node irradiation.
While it was wrong to thoughtlessly irradiate all patients, it is equally wrong to omit this adjuvant therapy for the whole group of patients. Again, the key is a carefully balanced selection of patients.

Side Effects of Radiotherapy of the Breast

Sequelae of radiotherapy are related to the organs encompassed in the treatment volume, and to the dose given. The time at which the radiation effects are seen is dependent on the cell turnover time of the irradiated tissues.
The tissues which are always irradiated are the skin and the breast tissue itself. The axilla

with the vascular and nervous plexus and the anterior mediastinum are only irradiated when the regional lymph nodes are treated.
The ribs and part of the lungs can sometimes be included in the treatment volume of the breast and always when irradiating the nodal regions.
The oesophagus should only receive moderate doses when using appropriate techniques for the irradiation of parasternal nodes. Finally, irradiation of the heart should be avoided as much as possible, which is feasible with modern techniques but which was very often not done in old treatments.
The main effect of irradiation is inhibition of the proliferation of cells. This means that in tissues needing continuous proliferation, side effects will be seen rapidly, a few weeks after the start of therapy, during radiotherapy or in the period immediately afterwards. This is the case for instance for skin, gastrointestinal mucosa and the haematopoietic system. Immediately at the start of irradiation some (transient) erythema and oedema of the breast can occur. The true epidermal reactions of the skin start only after two to three weeks. With the high-energy equipment used nowadays, which spares superficial layers, epidermitis usually remains limited to a dry desquamation, except in skin folds (inframammary fold and axilla) where limited moist desquamation can occur. This heals normally within a few weeks.
Reactions of the oesophageal mucosa usually start slightly earlier (second week) and can lead to some dysphagia but can be limited by techniques limiting the dose to the oesophagus (e.g., using electrons for part of the treatment of the parasternal nodes).
Decreases in the values of blood cells can occur, in relation to the volume of ribs and vertebrae irradiated, but are rare.
In the weeks and months after irradiation a period of radiation pneumonitis can develop, either silently or with a period of coughing. Also some periostitis around the ribs can occur with a tenderness which often causes some worry to the patients who think the pain comes from the breast itself.
Late side effects come predominantly from connective tissue and small vascular structures. After high doses, a slowly progressive fibrosis can develop in the breast, which can be continuous over several years. Small abnormal vessels can be formed, called telangiectasia, but usually only after very high doses. This starts only after two years and can progress until five years or longer after treatment.
One of the frequent complications from earlier treatment periods was arm oedema. This was fairly frequent when very extensive surgery (Halsted procedure with radical axillary dissection) was combined with postoperative radiotherapy. The better selection of procedures with the definition of a group of "inoperable" patients, the less radical surgical procedures and more sophisticated irradiation procedures have led to the disappearance of the invalidating, pronounced arm oedema. A relatively small group of patients still has some, limited, oedema, usually without clinical repercussions.

Palliative Irradiation of Metastatic Disease

Breast tumours are fairly radiosensitive. This means that symptoms from distant localisations can often rapidly be relieved by irradiation. As a number of breast tumours grow slowly such effects can often be long lasting and contribute greatly to the comfort of the patient.
When the diagnosis of metastases is made in breast cancer the treatment objective becomes palliation. Therapy options are radiotherapy for well defined tumour volumes, and systemic treatment, hormonal as well as cytotoxic.
Decisions in palliative therapy are often more difficult to make than in curative situations as they require a careful balancing of all these factors with also a comparison of expected benefit and side effects of therapy. One of the basic principles to be respected in this situation is that not all localisations have to be treated, but only those which are symptomatic, those which can be expected to become so in the near future, or those which carry the risk of serious complications.
The most frequent objectives for palliative radiotherapy in breast cancer are skeletal metastases. A few basic rules can be given. Painful and osteolytic lesions should usually

be irradiated when this is possible volumewise. For weight-bearing bones (vertebrae, femora) the decision to irradiate is taken earlier than for other bones (skull, os ilium) as the risk for complication is greater. The risk of fracture should always be reduced maximally by preventive irradiation as the recovery from a pathological fracture is much slower than from an osteolysis. Osteoblastic lesions are usually only treated when painful. Imminent vertebral fractures or actual collapses should be considered as medical emergencies. Finally, the dose to be selected is dependent on the prognosis of the disease. There is no use in giving long treatments and high doses to patients with a very short expected survival time. However, for solitary lesions, late relapses and slow growing tumours, it is worthwhile to conduct carefully planned treatments in order to obtain long remissions with minimal late side effects.
The other classical situations in which radiotherapy can often be a very useful palliative agent are nodal relapses, in the primary lymph node areas as well as in others, cutaneous localisations and brain metastases.
The nodal localisations often lead to symptoms of compression in blood and lymph vessels, or in other tracti such as respiratory or gastrointestinal. Rapid relief is usually possible if treatment is carried out early enough.
Skin localisations are a psychological burden to the patient and often cause hygienic problems. Due to their location they can usually be irradiated with a minimal burden for surrounding tissues (electrons).
Finally for brain metastases, the decision to treat can sometimes be complex. For the patient who has not yet received chemotherapy, the resulting alopecia is a burden. The potential consequences of other localisations, the still available therapeutic tools with systemic therapy and the overall prognosis will play an important role in the decision making process.
In conclusion, it should emphatically be stated that the patient who cannot be cured can still be treated with very good results. Decisions on symptom relief are difficult but good palliation is a medical success, greatly contributing to the patient's quality of life. Errors in palliation, both undertreatment and overtreatment, are medical errors, just as much as shortcomings in curative treatment. Palliation in breast cancer requires a multidisciplinary approach. Radiotherapy plays an important role in this aspect of treatment.

Adjuvant Systemic Therapy

More than half of the women rendered disease free after treatment of the primary tumour eventually develop overt metastases. Metastatic breast cancer is an incurable condition and the majority of patients will have to live with symptoms related to the site of the metastases, and will die of complications related to its progression. This reality was the basis for the development of therapies aimed at reducing relapses and, hence, mortality of patients who were clinically disease free as a result of surgery. The basic hypotheses for the use of a systemic treatment are:

- ❏ In those patients who will eventually relapse, microscopic disease is already present at diagnosis.
- ❏ Cytotoxic or endocrine therapies which have proven to be active in advanced disease (leading to tumour shrinkage) should also have an effect upon such a small tumour cell burden.
- ❏ The methods of primary tumour ablation have little effect upon survival.

There Is No "Magic Bullet"

The effects of adjuvant systemic therapies upon survival are modest, and it is necessary to conduct randomised trials to show these treatments are more effective in controlling disease than tumour ablation alone.
It is therefore essential that certain issues be clarified before results from randomised trials in breast cancer can be interpreted or a cost-benefit analysis performed for patient-care purposes.
The magnitude of the effect of therapy in terms of reduced relapses is estimated at about 30%-35% within 5 years. This also means that 65%-70% of the patients who are estimated to relapse will do so despite treatment.
The magnitude of the effect of therapy in terms of reduced mortality is estimated at about 20%-25% within 5 years. This also means that 75%-80% of the patients who die will do so despite therapy.
The relative risk of relapse or death is the most important factor for appreciation of the real impact of therapy upon a population. A group of patients with few positive lymph nodes, which might have an estimated 5-year 40% relapse rate, will reduce this risk to "only" 25% if treated. The issue for a population with well differentiated, small tumours and no axillary node involvement is different. For these patients a 5-year relapse percentage might be 10% or less and the best available treatment will not reduce by more than 3%-4% the estimated prognosis at that time point. This latter population is not frequently observed and therefore the issue of defining the threshold for overtreatment is matter of controversy. It is important to understand that the only way to solve this controversy is to develop more effective therapies, and the only way to do so is to offer the patients a treatment within the framework of a clinical trial. Unless, that is, the legendary "magic bullet" should be found.

Best Available Systemic Treatments

Review of the literature and, especially, the meta-analysis or overview, a new method for pooling results from all available randomised trials, were very useful for highlighting those therapies which, for a given population, were found to bestow real benefit in terms of disease-free survival or overall survival.

Results of the first overview of randomised clinical trials were recently published, and the effects of adjuvant tamoxifen (Tam) and of prolonged cytotoxic therapy (CT) on mortality are summarised in Table 1.
Based upon available results the following remarks regarding the treatment of patients can be made.

Premenopausal Patients

(also defined as 50 years old or younger)

The majority of the studies were carried out in patients with metastatic axillary nodes (N+). Retrospective analyses of the ultimate effect of therapy in subpopulations defined by the number of nodes involved suggest that patients with a large number of metastatic nodes have a very bad prognosis, also if treated. New treatment modalities are required for this population.
The effects of adjuvant chemotherapy are not dependent upon the presence and concentration of steroid hormone receptor content in the primary tumour. The response of this population to an endocrine therapy might depend upon steroid hormone receptor content, but both issues (i.e., endocrine therapy for premenopausal women and the role of hormone receptors with regard to its use) are controversial.
The most frequently studied regimen of combination chemotherapy with cyclophosphamide, methotrexate and 5-fluorouracil (CMF), given for the duration of at least 6 months, was found to reduce early mortality by about 25%. The combination is more effective than a single agent therapy (alkylating agents such as melphalan or cyclophosphamide, alone).

Table 1. Reduction in annual odds of death (% ± S.D) by age

Treatment	Any age	<50 yrs	> 50 yrs
CT vs No CT	14 ± 4	22 ± 6	4 ± 5
PolyCT vs No CT	17 ± 5	26 ± 7	8 ± 6
Tam vs No Tam	16 ± 3	-1 ± 8	20 ±3
> 2 years Tam vs No Tam	19 ± 4	1 ± 9	23 ± 4

Details related to adjuvant systemic therapies with some emphasis upon characteristics of the patient population:
The duration of treatment with available combinations should be approximately 6 months. One cycle of perioperative therapy, although having some beneficial effect upon outcome, is not enough.
The intensity of the therapy in terms of administered cytotoxic dose is likely to play an important role in achieving optimal antitumour effects. Prospective studies will show whether this hypothesis, based upon theoretical and experimental models as well as retrospective analyses of trials, is real.
The timing of cytotoxic treatment is theoretically very important. Early administration has been hypothesised to avert the establishment of resistance of tumour cells to therapy. The very early start of treatment failed to provide an advantage in terms of outcome in comparison with the usual delay (4-5 weeks after surgery).
Another aspect of timing of therapy is related to attempts to overcome resistance. The observation that patients who relapsed after cessation of adjuvant chemotherapy and prolonged disease-free survival nevertheless respond to the same drug regimen indicates that initial resistance to the therapy might be reversible. Late reintroduction of adjuvant therapy is being investigated.
The use of drug regimens containing other drugs known to be very effective in advanced disease is the subject of many studies. It is unclear today whether an adriamycin-containing regimen will significantly improve outcome as compared to the CMF-type therapy. Clarification of the issue awaits results from ongoing trials.
Oophorectomy or radiation-induced castration has been shown to reduce relapse and to prolong survival. However, these effects of therapy did not reach statistical significance in most of the trials, and appeared only after a long follow-up time. The role of castration was also questioned in relation to the use of chemotherapy: cytotoxic drug-induced amenorrhoea was associated with a better outcome, especially for patients with oestro-

gen receptor-rich tumours. Whether this endocrine manipulation provides some of the beneficial effects of the cytotoxic drug regimen is unclear. It is likely that chemotherapy is effective primarily via a direct cytocidal effect on tumour cells, but that some of the effects are mediated via hormonal ablation. Prospective studies comparing endocrine therapies with cytotoxic regimens are ongoing.
The effects of a prolonged endocrine therapy (for 2 years or more) employing the antioestrogen tamoxifen in premenopausal women have not been extensively investigated. Its use for this patient population is controversial, also because the overview which was conducted of all available trials did not provide conclusive evidence. Some large trials, especially a recent one in patients with N-negative disease and oestrogen receptor-positive primaries, have shown early benefit in terms of disease-free survival. Only one trial, carried out comparing tamoxifen with a CMF combination chemotherapy, showed a significant advantage in favour of the latter (see also details on the treatment of N-negative patients). Results from ongoing studies should expand the present knowledge about this issue as well.

Postmenopausal Patients

Most of the trials were conducted in patients with N-positive disease. The steroid hormone receptor content of the primary tumour seems to relate to response to endocrine therapy, although this issue, too, is controversial.
A prolonged treatment (2 years or more) with the antioestrogen tamoxifen has been shown to reduce early mortality by about 20%. There is no convincing evidence that a combination chemotherapy (e.g., CMF) is of equal or better efficacy than tamoxifen for the postmenopausal patient population.
Details related to adjuvant systemic therapies with some emphasis upon characteristics of the patient population:
The duration of treatment with tamoxifen should exceed 2 years. Preliminary evaluations of trials which compare shorter with longer duration appear to indicate an advantage for the prolonged administration. There is some concern related to the observation of an excess of endometrial cancer under prolonged treatment. This has still to be confirmed, but serves as a good example of the uncertainty related to late treatment effects in breast cancer.
The doses of tamoxifen which have been used in many trials range between 20 and 40 mg/day. The 20 mg dose is reasonable, and there is no data which favours the use of higher doses.
A combined chemo- and endocrine therapy (tamoxifen and a CMF-type regimen) resulted in a significantly improved outcome as compared to the endocrine therapy alone given for the same duration (one year). The role of the combination is therefore unclear and awaits results from studies which compare initial chemotherapy followed by prolonged tamoxifen.
Evidence from trials in patients with node-negative disease show that the effect of endocrine therapy in terms of disease-free survival is significant, especially for those with oestrogen receptor-positive primaries. Other studies in which selected patients were included (large tumours or only oestrogen receptor-negative tumours) showed a significant effect of chemotherapy, which was of a magnitude similar to that observed for node-positive breast cancer (see also details on the treatment of N-negative patients).
Treatment of an elderly population (65-80 years of age) has been the subject of very few trials; endocrine therapy with tamoxifen improved disease-free survival in this postmenopausal population.
Other forms of endocrine therapies (e.g., aminoglutethimide, medroxyprogesterone acetate) which were investigated in a small number of patients, were associated with a significant amount of toxicity and no apparent advantage upon the lesser toxic endocrine therapy.

Therapy of Patients with N-Negative Disease

Until recently patients with no metastatic involvement of the ipsilateral axillary lymph nodes were excluded from trials investigating adjuvant therapies for breast cancer. This was due to the data available which indicated this form of presentation of the disease at the lowest risk for relapse. Younger observations, especially the definition of some prognostic variables (e.g., tumour size, oestrogen receptor content in the primary tumour, labelling index, DNA content, S-phase fraction, etc.), provided convincing evidence that some patients with N-negative disease have a higher chance of relapse. Trials which specifically relate to the question of adjuvant systemic therapy for a selected or unselected population of patients (selection by oestrogen receptor content or by tumour size) are displayed in Table 2. All trials are surgically controlled. The NSABP (National Surgical Adjuvant Breast Project) trial B-14 is also placebo controlled.

The impact of the disease-free survival benefit upon overall survival is yet unknown, and the risk of overtreating this patient population by offering adjuvant therapy to all, is real. Therapy for patients with N-negative disease should best be considered within the framework of clinical trials.

Side Effects of Adjuvant Systemic Therapy

CMF-type combination chemotherapy: The cytotoxic effects of a chemotherapy regimen may be reflected by the blood cell counts. Thus, monitoring of the cellular components of the blood represents the routine evaluation of patients who receive such a therapy. Leukopenia should virtually be an inevitable effect of each course of treatment. Its nadir values are important for determination of the subsequent dose.

Table 2. Results of controlled trials on adjuvant systemic therapy

Trial, name of group or institution (Treatment)	Selection of patients	No. of patients	Years of reported follow-up	Results in disease-free survival (%) TREATED	CONTROLS
OSAKO (LMF)	No	121	9	63	60
Midlands (LMF)	No	543	5	75	74
Mainz (CMF)	No	175	5	82	72
Wien (CMFV)	No	128	5	86	78
Milano (i.v.CMF)	ER-neg	90	5	87	45
NSABP B-13 (M+F+Leucovorin)	ER-neg	741	4	80	71
NSABP B-14 (Tamoxifen)	ER-pos	2644	4	82	77
Intergroup 0011 (CMF)	ER-neg, (ER-pos if T > 3 cm)	422	3	84	67
Ludwig V (perioperative CMF)	No	1275	4	77	73

Table 3 lists the most common side effects of a cyclophosphamide, methotrexate and 5-fluorouracil combination chemotherapy, and some relevant remarks.
Other side effects of rare occurrence include hepatotoxicity (methotrexate), cutaneous rash (methotrexate and 5-fluorouracil), ataxia (5-fluorouracil) and phlebitis.
Depression and anxiety related to the treatment are less common than is generally believed. A constant flow of information to the patient and to her family is needed to reinforce coping efforts.
Tamoxifen therapy: the use of this drug is associated with a very low incidence of side effects. The most frequent are hot flushes and epigastric discomfort, especially in the first weeks of therapy. Tolerance eventually improves so that discontinuation of the drug is required in only very few cases. Theoretically, hypercalcaemia can appear after treatment start, due to the slight oestrogenic effect of the drug.
Some caution is required in the treatment of premenopausal women: the drug induces ovulation. Furthermore, prolonged administration was associated with increased oestrogen levels.

Table 3. Most common side effects of cyclophosphamide, methotrexate and 5-fluorouracil combination

Side effect	Incidence	Remarks
Leukopenia	70-100%	Due to all three drugs, usually appears between the 9th-21st day of the chemotherapy cycle. If severe requires supportive care (against infections and other associated complications). Avoid salicylates, sulphonamides, etc., which might increase toxic effects of methotrexate. (*)
Thrombo-cytopenia	20-40%	Might be severe in 5% of the cases and, if so, should be treated.
Nausea, vomiting, epigastric pain	60-80%	May be controlled by a proper antiemetic therapy. An antiemetic programme must be discussed with the patient before the first course to avoid conditioning.
Stomatitis, mucositis, diarrhoea	20-30%	Mainly due to methotrexate and 5-fluorouracil. Oral hygiene should be intensified prophylactically. Antimycotic agents should be used when present. Hydration must be guaranteed. Avoid continuation of cytotoxic drugs until recovery. (*)
Conjunctivitis	10-15%	Should be treated with medication (if no infection, use topical hydrocortisone).
Alopecia	50-75%	Prepare patient psychologically; advise hair dresser prior to loss of hair since 25-30% will require a wig. Some avoidance of severe hair loss may be achieved by scalp cooling used during all i.v. drug regimens.
Cystitis	10-15%	Haemorrhagic, due to cyclophosphamide. To avoid it the patient should maintain high fluid intake. May be treated with mesna.

Table 4. Common adjuvant systemic therapy regimens

CMF regimen: repeat cycle every 28 days

Cyclophosphamide	100 mg/m2	orally	Days 1-14
Methotrexate	40 mg/m2	i.v.	Days 1 and 8
5-Fluorouracil	600 mg/m2	i.v	Days 1 and 8

For duration of the treatment see text

CMF regimen: repeat cycle every 21 days

Cyclophosphamide	600 mg/m2	i.v	Day 1
Methotrexate	40 mg/m2	i.v.	Day 1
5-Fluorouracil	600 mg/m2	i.v.	Day 1

For duration of the treatment see text

Tamoxifen

The drug is administered orally, continuously, at a dosage of 20 mg/day

Treatment of Overt Metastatic Disease

Almost 90% of the patients are diagnosed as having operable disease. The term operable refers to the fact that the disease is confined to the mammary gland and to the ipsilateral axilla. The majority of this population will relapse, commonly in regions which are distant from the first site of the tumour. Data available after a long-term follow-up (of 31 years) show that metastatic disease may appear at any time after a successful treatment of the primary tumour. Overt metastatic disease must, with very few exceptions, be considered an incurable condition. The patient who relapses will eventually die with or of metastatic breast cancer. The majority of the patients who relapse will require palliation of symptoms of metastatic disease, and at such time the attitude toward the patient should take into account some quality-of-life considerations. Ideally the therapy for metastatic disease with the available treatments should obtain the maximal relief of symptoms (possibly even start therapy just before their onset), for the maximal duration with the minimal burden of side effects. The decision to treat and the choice of treatment must therefore take into account the extent of the disease and the related symptoms, not only those which are present but also those likely to occur within a short period of time. The objective is to increase the total duration of time with no or few disease-related symptoms. The choice of treatment must also take into consideration certain biological features which define the aggressiveness of the disease:

❑ shorter disease-free interval (the time period between the first surgery and the onset of overt metastatic disease);
❑ multiple organ involvement (bone, liver, lung, subcutaneous tissue are each to be considered as one organ involvement); the extent of damage to the organ involved is very important: jaundice or thrombocytopenia due to massive liver or bone marrow metastases, respectively, are indications of a dire prognosis;
❑ low or no steroid hormone receptors in the tumour tissue (because of greater chance of longer responses obtainable with hormonal manipulation);
these are the most important factors in defining a significantly shorter survival.

Additional host-related factors are best objectively quantified by :

❑ performance status (measured for example, on a scale of 5 grades, which indicates the extent to which the patient is hampered by the disease, e.g., zero indicates a fully active patient, while 4 indicates a 100% bed-ridden person); the sicker the patient, the worse the prognosis.
❑ prior adjuvant therapy, especially if completed shortly before the appearance of metastases, is associated with a dire prognosis.

Therapies, Choice and Conduct

The choice of the type of treatment is largely dependent upon the subjective attitudes of the physician and the patient toward any therapeutic manoeuvre. In certain circumstances radiation or surgery might be useful (see paragraph on therapeutic issues related to special sites of overt metastases). In most instances a systemic therapy is required to control all disease manifestations. The subjective factors related to the choice of treatment, particularly chemotherapy, have their impact mainly because of the absence of curative prospects at the metastatic phase of the disease. Personal attitude rather than data from clinical trials dictates the treatment

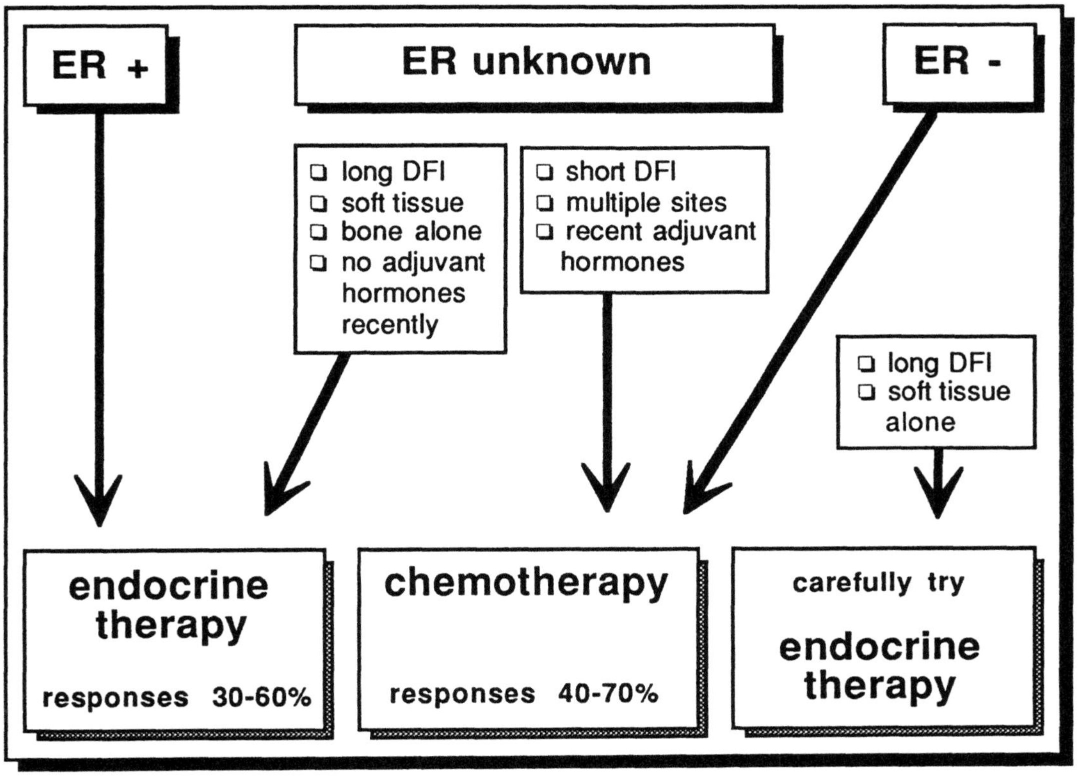

choice when quality-of-life issues are considered. It is recommended that the therapeutic approach based primarily upon the oestrogen receptor status of the disease be chosen, especially if this was determined from metastatic tissue. Features which indicate the aggressivity or presumed chronic (i.e., slower) course of the disease (disease-free interval, site and number of metastases, and the history of prior adjuvant therapy) must also be considered. The therapeutic approach for selection of initial treatment of overt metastatic disease is displayed in the figure.

Endocrine Therapy

Oophorectomy: surgical, or in some instances radiation-induced. Indicated for premenopausal women.
The strategic role of drug-induced castration (LA-RH superanalogues) is not yet established.

Antioestrogens:
Tamoxifen administered orally in a dosage of 20 mg a day, continuously.

Progestins:
Medroxyprogesterone acetate 500-1000 mg orally, daily;
Megestrol acetate 160 mg orally, daily.

Androgens:
Fluoxymestrone acetate 30 mg orally, daily.

Aromatase inhibitors:
Aminoglutethimide 250 mg orally, 2-4 times daily, together with hydrocortisone replacement, 40 mg daily, in divided doses.

The first reported endocrine therapy for inoperable breast cancer was surgical oophorectomy to control locally advanced disease.
Subsequently, other surgical manipulations

directed towards suppression of steroid hormone production (adrenalectomy, hypophysectomy) were used. These latter were abandoned due to developments in endocrinological pharmacology.
Research into steroid hormones and the subsequent discovery of oestrogens, androgens and progestins, followed by anti-oestrogens and aromatase-inhibitors, and, recently, hormone-releasing analogues, have all been added to the arsenal of weapons which can be used for a reasonable palliation of patients with metastatic breast cancer.
The response rate to endocrine therapy of an unselected population is estimated to range between 20% and 40%, and response rates for patients selected on the basis of oestrogen receptor content in their tumours range between 40% and 60%. Even patients with unfavourable sites of metastatic disease respond to endocrine therapy if they are selected on the basis of a high oestrogen-receptor content of the tumour.

The following remarks regarding the use of endocrine therapies derive from common medical experience and results from randomised studies conducted in this field:

❑ The time to response to endocrine therapy is usually 6 or more weeks. Assessment of the clinical situation of the patient must allow for this time lag.
❑ Tamoxifen is considered a first-line therapy. Comparison of this drug with other endocrine treatments, with mainly oestrogens, androgens, progestins and surgical ablation, show a similar efficacy for them. The benefit from tamoxifen is impressive in terms of its dearth of side effects.
❑ Progestins or aromatase inhibitors should be considered a valid secondary endocrine therapy. Response to the primary hormonal therapy indicates a chance of about 30% to 50% of obtaining a response to a subsequent therapy.
❑ Combination of endocrine therapies did not show a significant advantage over using the agents sequentially. The only hormonal combination therapy which was shown to improve results was the one with tamoxifen and prednisone.

Chemotherapy

Traditionally, the use of cytotoxic agents was considered for all patients whose young age or aggressive disease impressed the physician as requiring a rapid, objective tumour regression. The majority of the drug combinations today may be used at any age, provided there are no important organ function impairments (i.e., normal renal, liver and bone marrow functions).
Overall response rates to chemotherapy are reported to range between 43% and 82% with a certain proportion classified as complete (the latter range from anecdotal to 1/4 of the patients). The median time to response is said to range between 7 and 14 weeks, although initial response associated with a reasonable palliation may already start after 1-3 weeks. The median duration of response to drug combinations ranges from 6 months to one year. Some patients are described as being in response for more than a decade. Definitive evidence concerning the impact of chemotherapy on overall survival is not available, but some does exist to indicate that any improvement in overall survival could be limited to patients with aggressive tumours as opposed to those with less rapidly progressing disease.

❑ Factors associated with increased response rates are: good performance status, limited number of tumour sites, and metastases in soft tissue alone.
❑ Prior response to endocrine therapy is a factor which is associated with a prolonged duration of response or survival.
❑ The steroid hormone receptor content in the tumour does not *per se* influence chemotherapy outcome.
❑ A decreased probability of response is described for patients with bone and liver metastases, prior radiation therapy or systemic adjuvant treatment, especially if recently terminated, or decreased lymphocyte counts.
The following indications for choice of the therapy are emerging from the results of many clinical trials:

Table 1. Common combinations used in metastatic breast cancer

Regimen	Dose	Route	Schedule
CMF (P)			Repeat q 28 days
C	100 mg/m2	p.o.	days 1-14
M	40 mg/m2	i.v.	days 1 and 8
F	600 mg/m2	i.v.	days 1 and 8
(P)	40 mg/m2	p.o.	days 1-14
I.V. CMF			Repeat q 21 days
C	600 mg/m2	i.v.	day 1
M	40 mg/m2	i.v.	day 1
F	600 mg/m2	i.v.	day 1
LMF (p)			Repeat q 28 days
L	5 mg/m2	p.o.	days 1-14
M	40 mg/m2	i.v.	days 1 and 8
F	600 mg/m2	i.v.	days 1 and 8
(p) low-dose	12.5 mg	p.o.	days 1-14
AC			Repeat q 21-28 days
A	40 mg/m2	i.v.	day 1
C	200 mg/m2	p.o.	day 3-6
CAF			Repeat q 3 weeks
C	400-500 mg/m2	i.v.	day 1
A	40-50 mg/m2	i.v	day 1
F	400-500 mg/m2	i.v.	days 1 and 8

C= cyclophosphamide; M= methotrexate; F= 5-fluorouracil; L=chlorambucil (Leukeran™); A= adriamycin, doxorubicin

❑ A combination chemotherapy yielded a higher response rate than single-agent therapy in almost all trials which have compared the two. The combination should therefore be considered first. Exceptions relate to the use of cyclophosphamide and adriamycin, which are also considered the most active drugs in the treatment of breast cancer.

❑ Alternation of non-cross-resistant drug combinations with available agents, including cyclophosphamide and adriamycin, did not appear to influence survival.

❑ The use of adriamycin-containing regimens has been associated with higher response rates and response duration (and even with some overall survival advantage for certain subgroups with particularly aggressive forms of disease) than have the "standard" methotrexate-based combinations (methotrexate-based regimens administered weekly were found to be equivalent to adriamycin-based combinations). The sequential use of adriamycin-containing regimens and methotrexate combinations is a common oncological procedure. New anthracyclines (4-epi-adriamycin and mitoxantrone) were found to be less toxic than their older relative and also slightly less effective.

❑ High-dose chemotherapy: The assumption that high-dose chemotherapy would probably induce more response and, hence, more efficiently palliate more patients and perhaps prolong survival, is a subject of controversy. An increased complete remission rate has been observed with the use of this intensive treatment modality, but it remains unclear whether this will have an impact upon survival. New dose-intensity investigations will be conducted in the near future, made possible by the availability of colony-stimulating-factors (CSFs) and the autologous bone marrow technology.

❑ Combined chemo-endocrine therapy: Since breast cancer is believed to contain two distinct populations of malignant cells - one hormone-sensitive and the other hormone-resistant - efforts have been made to influence the growth of both by combining chemo- and endocrine therapies. While the combination has yielded higher response rates, there has been no advantage in terms of survival. In postmenopausal patients it has become clear that the sequential use of the two modalities confers a therapeutic advantage, especially in patients with slow-growing metastases. Among premenopausal women there might be a population with particularly aggressive tumours which will benefit from the combination, but selection of such a group is controversial.

❑ Secondary treatments: Once the first sequence of treatment combinations has been proven to be insufficient for controlling the disease and especially its symptoms, a "salvage" treatment regimen might include mitomycin-C and vinblastin.

Response to Systemic Treatment and its Impact upon Patients: Quality-of-Life Issues

The practice of measuring response rates for selecting treatments for patients in whom the principal therapeutic objective is palliation is questionable. Some evidence indicates that, indeed, objective response and subjective palliation obtained by chemotherapy are correlated. Patients who respond objectively to treatment tend also to improve significantly. Furthermore, about 33% of the patients who do not respond have some degree of palliation, especially relief of pain.

While objective measurement of response might be important for finding an active drug or drug regimen, evaluation of the impact of therapy on the quality of the patients' lives requires a more subjective definition. There have been attempts to have the patient define her symptoms, the side effects of the drugs, her anxiety and depression, personal relationships, physical performance, sense of well-being and efforts to cope with the disease and its symptoms. In one such instance the objective was to answer the question of whether chemotherapy may be interrupted once a remission has been obtained and resumed only upon progression. The trial compared this intermittent regimen to a continuous therapy regimen. Patients on the intermittent drug regimen had a slightly shorter survival, but, unexpectedly, those on the continuous regimen documented a better perception of their well-being. It is essential that future trials include studies of the quality of life.

Therapeutic Issues Related to Special Sites of Overt Metastases

The choice of treatment of overt metastatic disease very often depends on a set of specific clinical problems almost exclusively related to the site. The data which serve as a basis for selection of a particular approach are typically derived from observations and clinical experience (rather than from controlled trials). The most frequent metastatic conditions are :

❑ Local recurrence including scar and ipsilateral axilla: surgery is usually applied if the recurrence is circumscribed. Radiation therapy is applied as adjuvant to surgery and in instances when the excision could not be radical. The roles of adjuvant chemo- and endocrine therapies are being investigated in clinical trials.

❑ Breast recurrence after a breast-conserving procedure (QUART or lumpectomy, axillary clearance and local radiation therapy. Usually a mastectomy is performed. The role of adjuvant systemic therapies is being investigated.

❑ Contralateral breast relapse. The prognosis of the patient with appearance of a new (or metastatic) node in the contralateral breast does not worsen the prognosis of the patient, provided that the factors related to the second neoplasia do not indicate that the tumour behaves more aggressively. The situation is similar when the two tumours appear simultaneously. The approach to the patient must be with curative intent and a local therapy appropriate for the extent of the disease (mastectomy and axillary clearance, or a breast-conserving procedure) applied. The role of adjuvant systemic therapy has not been studied.

❑ Metastatic disease in the bone alone. This is usually a disease which will have a prolonged course. Systemic therapy is usually required, but irradiation for localised pain, and surgery for weight-bearing and functionally important structures should be regularly discussed. The use of biphosphonates, compounds which arrest bone destruction by inhibiting osteoclasts, has been defined. The manner of their administration (route, schedule and duration) await data from ongoing studies.

❑ Brain metastases. Usually the symptoms are associated with peritumoral oedema. Steroid therapy (e.g., dexamethasone 16 mg/day divided into 4 doses) is usually associated with a rapid improvement of symptoms. Radiation therapy follows. The role of surgery for isolated and accessible metastasis is undefined. The roles of systemic therapy or regional chemotherapy are being investigated.

❑ Spinal cord compression. Its onset represents an emergency and the damage must be immediately defined. Treatment with high-dose dexamethasone should precede even the myelographic evaluation of the site of the compression. In general, a tumour-dependent compression may be approached with a primary radiation therapy. A bone fracture-dependent lesion, especially with bone fragments which might cause part of the neurological damage, is an indication for primary surgery.

❑ Symptomatic malignant effusions (pleural, pericardial). An attempt to improve symptoms by drainage is usually followed by instillation of compounds which include tetracyclines, cytotoxic drugs such as bleomycin (prior radiation therapy and renal function impairment enhance the toxic effects of this drug), thiotepa, adriamycin and "biological response modifiers" (such as a suspension of corynebacterium parvum). Persistence of a symptomatic effusion might require the more extensive surgical intervention of pleurectomy or pericardial stripping.

Summary

The therapy for patients with overt metastatic breast cancer must be selected for its efficacy in providing palliation. The decision to treat and the choice of treatment must be made in view of the extent of the disease and its related symptoms, as well as other parameters which might be predictive of response to the least toxic therapy. However, the target of planning individual treatment programmes with a sequence of therapies designed to provide the best palliation with available means, is difficult to reach, primarily because of the heterogeneity of the disease and the dearth of experience in assessing the quality of life. In so far as possible, palliation should be carried out in the patient's own environment, and the treating team, including the family physician, should endeavour to approximate the target as nearly as possible by coordinating their activities.

Rehabilitation

Rehabilitation after breast cancer treatment has become easier than in the past, as the iatrogenic effects of breast cancer therapies today are much slighter. However, modern rehabilitation units have increasingly investigated the delicate psychological mechanisms which are connected with breast cancer. It has been said that diagnosis of breast cancer may represent an overwhelming human crisis for the patient, for her family and also for her doctor. The rehabilitation process must, therefore, consider any physical damage to be corrected within the setting of this human crisis.

Early iatrogenic effects are: 1) capsular articular symptoms, as a result of a scapulohumeral block due to positioning of the upper limb and insufficient postoperative arm motion, 2) lesion of the long thoracic nerve. This lesion produces the so-called "winged scapula" syndrome, which, however, disappears spontaneously in the majority of cases; 3) lesion of the intercostobrachial nerve. This lesion is very frequent and often unavoidable when performing correct axillary dissection. It generally produces anaesthesia and paraesthesia in the ventral aspect of the proximal portion of the upper limb.

Late iatrogenic results are mainly lymphoedema of the arm and lesions of the brachial plexus.

Lymphoedema is much less frequent today than in the past due to modified surgical techniques and the abandonment of postoperative RT on the axilla. It is present in 5%-10% of patients who have undergone surgery, but the very serious cases are no more than 2%-3%. The aetiology of lymphoedema is the removal of the axillary nodes and the factors which increase the risk are infection, venous thrombosis, haematoma, tension of the flaps. Another important factor is recurrent lymphangitis of the arm. Lymphoedema can be avoided first by accurate axillary surgery and then by early movement and physiotherapy. Treatment of lymphoedema consists of mechanical drainage (uniform or differentiated pneumatic pumps), manual drainage (massage and lymph drainage), the application of containing and compressing bandages and supports. An important component is a diet therapy, as an excess of calories due to intake of animal fats and animal protein increases the lymphoedema, whilst a loss of weight with an appropriate balanced diet generally obtains immediate reduction of the lymphoedema. Surgical treatment by lymphovenous anastomosis may give some satisfactory results.

Brachial plexus lesions are mainly due to the late effects of radiotherapy delivered in excessive doses to the supraclavicular fossa. The symptoms are generally progressive and may start with pain, hypo-aesthesia and paraesthesia proceeding to varying degrees of paresis. The roots mainly involved are C7, C8 and T1. Oedema of the arm frequently accompanies the paresis.

Very little can be done to reduce the great discomfort of the brachial plexus lesions. However, some results have been obtained with surgical neurolysis, or with hyperbaric oxygen therapy.

Rehabilitation programmes must consider the psychological aspects of the patients and the conditions of anxiety, anguish and depression which may be present in varying degrees. The fear of death, the fear of mutilation, the fear of isolation and the fear of pain are all components of the patients' psychological reactions. Information is the first step of rehabilitation and must be given to the patients before treatment. After surgery, individual mobilisation and group mobilisation are fundamental. Health care talks are important before discharging the patient so that she may be given all the necessary information for her follow-up. Discharged patients should be followed up and organised in groups for treatment with movement therapy and, finally, long-term individual therapy and family therapy may be required in specific cases.

Psychological Aspects

The psychological aspects of breast cancer have been extensively studied because they concern an organ which is closely associated with the sense of body image, with self-esteem, with femininity and sexuality. Furthermore, because breast cancer is so common, many women have already had secondary experience of the disease with a relative or friend who suffered a dire outcome. The factors which influence the psychological attitude of women upon impact with the diagnosis of breast cancer may be summarised as follows (modified from J.C. Holland):

Medical and Disease-Related Factors

❑ Stage of the disease at diagnosis.
❑ Prognostic factors other than stage (e.g., oestrogen-receptor content in the primary tumour), which might influence treatment choice.
❑ Type of primary treatment required: breast conservation, mastectomy, radiation, adjuvant chemotherapy.
❑ Psychological support by physician and staff.
❑ Availability of rehabilitation programmes.

Psychological and Psychosocial Factors

❑ Type and degree of influence upon life cycle tasks caused by the disease (e.g., presence of young children in the family, husband or partner, professional involvement).
❑ Ability to cope with stress.
❑ Prior psychiatric history.
❑ Availability of psychological and social support (partner, family, friends, self-help groups, etc.).

Sociocultural Factors, Treatment Options and Decision Making

❑ Changes in treatment options resulting from recently acquired knowledge (e.g., mastectomy vs breast conservation, radiation vs no radiation, chemotherapy vs endocrine therapy alone).
❑ Information from relatives and friends.
❑ Information from the popular press and media.
❑ Ethical imperative for patient participation in treatment choice.
❑ In some countries: legal imperative for knowledge of treatment options.
These factors underscore the complexity of the issues influencing the attitude of a woman to the disease.

Three broad psychosocial areas have been identified as related to the impact of breast cancer upon the patient:

❑ Psychological Discomfort:
Depression; Anxiety; Hostility.
❑ Changes in Life Patterns:
Physical discomfort;
Marital/Sexual Discomfort;
Reduced Activity Level;
Loss of Self-Esteem.
❑ Fears and Concern:
Cancer/Death;
Mastectomy/Mutilation.

The Psychosocial support of the patient should be directed toward each of these areas, and especially in the following instances:

❑ Pre-diagnosis and diagnosis phase:
Relieve anxiety by giving specific information about treatment options.

❑ Post-surgical phase:
Give information about prognosis and about the possibilities of improving it by available treatment options. Indicate the availability of a self-help group to testify to long term survival.

❑ Going/Coming home:
Help the patient in the logistics of rehabilitation (e.g., choice of prosthesis). Encourage the family if necessary. Offer to talk to relatives, particularly to those who might need special support (e.g., children, especially daughters, partner).

❑ Follow-up:
Give information rapidly to reduce anxiety.

❑ Relapse:
For many patients the reappearance of the disease is extremely difficult to cope with. Helping to overcome this particular moment of disillusionment is essential. Many patients who primarily had satisfactory reactions may suffer a significant breakdown. Information to reduce anxiety in such situations must be particularly precise, although many physicians have great difficulties in relaying bad news.

The influence of psychosocial factors upon the quality of life of the patient is very important. Research in this field might lead to knowledge of how psychological features influence not only the quality of life and well-being of the woman with breast cancer, but also her survival.
The variables which influence the intensity and duration of the psychosocial burden on the woman with breast cancer are extremely complex, and it is important for her that these factors be identified. This will provide a better quality of care for the patient as well as the possibility of individual intervention to relieve concerns and increase the sense of well-being.

❑ Preexisting variables.
Patient characteristics:
- Value of physical appearance for the patient;
- Value of breast appearance;
- Age;
- Preoperative expectations.

Environmental factors:
- Quality of marital / sexual relationships;
- Presurgical preparation by the physician;
- Type of relationship with other close relatives (sister).

❑ Post-operative variables.
Coping styles:
- Denial and denial-related mechanisms;
- Search for causes (self-blame and projection of blame)

Environmental factors:
- Time since diagnosis;
- Availability of support from physician, partner or family, from other patients;
- Therapy after surgery (radiation or systemic therapies).

Special Issues Related to Specific Types of Events and Situations:

❑ Psychological evaluation of the type of local treatment:
More concern about the insult to body image (breast conservation) versus the need to divest herself of the disease and its primary organ (a more extensive surgical approach). Similar approach with the choice of immediate breast reconstruction versus late reconstruction: the former should be considered in the light of the patient's fears of radiation therapy.

❑ Psychosocial evaluation for explaining systemic therapy to the patient.
In general, approaching the patient with this information requires a significant adjustment, mainly because of the widespread prejudice against systemic therapy, particularly chemotherapy, which evokes the image of people who are terminally ill.
While for many patients endocrine therapy alone with tamoxifen will require very little psychological preparation and adjustment because of the exceptional tolerance to this drug, chemotherapy needs to be extensively discussed with the patient. The main side effects which require specific discussion and a significant amount of help in adjustment are: hair loss, nausea and vomiting, weight gain (which is frequently observed (50%) due to

increased food intake - perhaps as a mechanism for self-conviction of well-being, and to decreased physical activity).

Discussion with the patient to broaden her spectrum of expectation and thus her therapy-coping ability should involve not only the physician, but also the nurses and other members of the rehabilitation team, as well as educational material.

Participation in clinical trials is imperative for defining better treatments in this disease. Evaluation of the patient might include assessment of the feasibility of offering her an available trial as a treatment option. Greater social acceptance of trials as a form of therapy framework for a disease in which virtually all advances in treatment have occurred through this type of clinical research, might also improve the patient's comprehension of treatment information and reduce the devastating confusion to which patients with malignant diseases are exposed.

❏ Special psychological support for depression, severe anxiety and other coping disorders.

Psychiatric consultation is only rarely considered but should be routinely sought when the patient's distress does not respond to the "usual" supportive measures. Depression may be severe, but suicide is rare. Psychiatric support, together with pharmacological antidepressant therapy, is useful. Anxiolytic drugs should be used to control symptoms during the day time. Insomnia should be treated appropriately.

❏ Support of the family of the breast cancer patient. Husband and children, especially daughters, might need help. Some deterioration of the mother-child relationship due to the disease has been identified in about 1/8 of a studied series. Especially vulnerable are daughters who might require some help in terms of information and support for coping.

Groups for Breast Cancer Patients: Psychological and Educational Support

The difficulties which many patients with breast cancer encounter during each phase of the disease have been described. A variety of psychological interventions carried out by groups have been proven to be of help to the patients. Those include postsurgical rehabilitation groups, family groups, psychoeducational groups for continuing care, and groups for patients with metastatic and terminal illness.

Self-help groups: These are based upon the principle that people who have experienced a crisis or a threatening situation have a unique contribution to make to others who are also undergoing the same experience

Breast surgery rehabilitation group: Many patients feel the need to ask for information from other women who have had a similar experience in the past. Such a group of women, with the aid of professionals, will provide great help to patients with a recent trauma, rapidly correcting misinformation and misconceptions, which are so often reasons for suffering.

It is important for the physicians and other health workers to recognise the need for such patient-based structures. It is important that some form of feedback be created to provide, when needed, the opportunity for a reasonable and informative cooperation.

REFERENCES

Epidemiology

Boyle, P. Epidemiology of Breast Cancer. In Bailliere's Clinical Oncology, Breast Cancer, U Veronesi Ed. London, Bailliere Tindall, 1988, pp 1-57

Dupont WD, Page DL. Risk factors for breast cancer in women with proliferative breast disease. New England Journal of Medicine 1985, 312:146-151

Dupont WD, Page DL. Breast cancer risk associated with proliferative disease, age at first birth and a family history of breast cancer. American Journal of Epidemiology 1987, 125:769-779

Ewertz M, Duffy SW. Risk of Breast Cancer in Relation to Reproductive Factors in Denmark. British Journal of Cancer 1988, 58:99-104

Haenszel WM 'Migrant Studies' In: Schottenfeld D and Fraumeni JF (eds) 'Cancer Epidemiology and Prevention', WD Saunders, Philadelphia 1982

Horn PL, Thompson WD. Risk of contralateral breast cancer: associations with factors related to initial breast cancer. American Journal of Epidemiology 1988, 128:309-323

La Vecchia C, Negri E, Boyle P, DeCarli A (in press) Anthropometric Variables and Breast Cancer. Cancer Research

Modan B, Chetrit A, Alfandary E, Katz L. Increased risk of Breast Cancer after low-dose irradiation. Lancet 1989, 1(8639):629-631

Clinical Diagnosis

Ciatto S, Pacini P, Azzini V et al. Preoperative staging of primary breast cancer - a multicentric study. Cancer 1988, (61):1038-1040

Ciatto S, Rosselli Del Turco M, Pacini P et al. Early detection of breast cancer recurrences through periodic follow up: Is it useless? Tumori 1985, (71):325-329

Ciatto S. Breast cancer diagnosis. In Bailliere's Clinical Oncology, Breast Cancer, U Veronesi Ed. London, Bailliere Tindall, 1988, pp.155-173

Collette HJA, Day NE, Rombach JJ et al. Evaluation of screening for breast cancer in a non randomized study (The DOM Project) by means of a case control study. Lancet 1984, (i):1224-1226

Haagensen CD. Physician's role in the detection and diagnosis of breast disease. In "Diseases of the Breast", Haagensen CD ed., 2nd ed., W.B.Saunders Co., Philadelphia, 1971, p.99-146.

Palli D, Rosselli Del Turco M, Buiatti E et al. A case-control study of the efficacy of a non randomized breast cancer screening program in Florence (Italy). Int J Cancer 1986, (38):501-504

Shapiro S, Venet W, Strax P et al. Ten to fourteeen year effect of screening on breast cancer mortality. J Natl Cancer Inst 1982, (34):349-355.

Tabar L, Fageberg CJG, Gad A et al. Reduction of mortality from breast cancer after mass screening with mammography. Lancet 1985, (i):829-832.

Verbeek ALM, Hendriks JHCL, Holland R et al. Reduction of breast cancer mortality through mass screening with modern mammography: first results of the Nijmegen Project, 1975-1981. Lancet 1984, (i)1222-1224.

Surgery

Fisher B, Bauer M, Margolese R et al. Five-year results of a randomised clinical trial comparing total mastectomy and segmental mastectomy with or without radiation in the treatment of breast cancer. New Engl J Med 1985, 312: 665-673

Fisher B, Redmond C, Fisher E et al. Ten-year results of a randomised clinical trial comparing radical mastectomy and total mastectomy with or without radiation. New Engl J Med 1985, 312: 674-681

Harris JR, Hellman S, Henderson IC, Kinne DW (Eds). Breast Diseases. Philadelphia Lippincott Company, 1987

Lacour J, Le M, Canceres E et al. Radical mastectomy versus radical mastectomy plus internal mammary dissection. Ten-year results of an international co-operative trial in breast cancer. Cancer 1983, 51: 1941-43

Veronesi U, Saccozzi R, Del Vecchio M et al. Comparing radical mastectomy with quadrantectomy, axillary dissection, and radiotherapy in patients with small cancers of the breast. New Engl J Med 1981, 305: 6-11

Veronesi U. Treatment of primary breast carcinoma. In Bailliere's Clinical Oncology, Breast Cancer, U Veronesi Ed. London, Bailliere Tindall, 1988, pp.175-192

Veronesi U, Costa A, Veronesi P. Cancer of the breast . In Surgical Oncology, A European Handbook, U Veronesi Ed. Berlin, Springer-Verlag, 1989, pp.827-878

Radiotherapy

Pierquin B, Maylin C, Owen R, Otmezguine Y, Raynal L, Mueller W, Hannoun S. Radical radiation therapy of breast cancer. Int J Rad Oncol Biol Phys 1980, 6:17-25

Van Limbergen E, Van der Schueren E, Vantongelen C. Cosmetic evaluation of breast conserving treatment for breast cancer. I. Proposal of a scoring system. Radiotherapy and Oncology 1989, 16:159-67

Yarnold JR. Factors affecting the cosmetic result and the scoring of normal tissue damage. In: Primary treatment of breast cancer: alternatives to mastectomy, M Peckham and JS Tobias Ed. 1986, pp. 114-130

Van Limbergen E, Van den Bogaert W, Van der Schueren E, Rijnders A. Tumour excision and radiotherapy as primary treatment of breast cancer. Analysis of patients and treatment parameters and local control. Radiotherapy and Oncology 1987, 8:1-9

Bedwinek J. Adjuvant irradiation for early breast cancer. An on-going controversy. Cancer 1984, 53: 729-739

Adjuvant systemic therapy

Early Breast Cancer Trialists' Collaborative Group: Effects of adjuvant tamoxifen and of cytotoxic therapy on mortality in early breast cancer. An overview of 61 randomized trials among 28,896 women. N Engl J Med 1988, 319: 1681-1692

Henderson IC: Adjuvant systemic therapy for early breast cancer. Curr Probl Cancer 1987, 11: 125-207

Proceedings of the NIH Consensus Development Conference on Adjuvant Chemotherapy and Endocrine therapy for Breast Cancer . NCI Monographs 1986, 1; 1-159

Adjuvant Therapy for Early Breast Cancer (Reports and Editorials for Treatment of N- disease). New Engl J Med 320 1989, 473-496, and 525-529

Wilson AJ, Baum M. Treatment of occult metastases. In Bailliere's Clinical Oncology, Breast Cancer, U Veronesi Ed. London, Bailliere Tindall, 1988, pp193-214

Metastatic Disease

The Australian and New Zealand Breast Cancer Trials Group. A randomized trial in postmenpausal patients with advanced breast cancer comparing endocrine and cytotoxic therapy given sequentially or in combination. J Clin Oncol 1986, 4: 186-193

Smith IE : Recurrent Disease. In Breast Diseases. JR Harris, S Hellman, IC Henderson, DW Kinne Eds, Philadelphia Lippincott Company, 1987, pp369-384

Goldhirsch A, Gelber RD. Treatment of overt metastatic breast cancer. In Bailliere's Clinical Oncology, Breast Cancer, U Veronesi Ed. London, Bailliere Tindall, 1988, pp 215-230

Psychological Aspects

Meyerowitz BE. Psychosocial correlates of breast cancer and its treatment. Psychol Bull 87:108-126, 1980

Holland JC, Rowland JH. Psychological reactions to breast cancer and its treatment. In: Breast Diseases. JR Harris, S Hellman, IC Henderson, DW Kinne Eds, Philadelphia Lippincott Company, 1987, pp 632-647

GPSR Compliance

The European Union's (EU) General Product Safety Regulation (GPSR) is a set of rules that requires consumer products to be safe and our obligations to ensure this.

If you have any concerns about our products, you can contact us on ProductSafety@springernature.com

In case Publisher is established outside the EU, the EU authorized representative is:

Springer Nature Customer Service Center GmbH
Europaplatz 3
69115 Heidelberg, Germany

Batch number: 10684220

Printed by Printforce, the Netherlands